Recent Results in Cancer Research

Volume 209

More information about this series at http://www.springer.com/series/392

Wolfgang Walther
Editor

Current Strategies in Cancer Gene Therapy

Springer

Editor
Wolfgang Walther
Department of Translational Oncology
Experimental and Clinical Research Center,
Charité University Medicine Berlin and
Max-Delbrück-Center for Molecular
Medicine
Berlin
Germany

ISSN 0080-0015 ISSN 2197-6767 (electronic)
Recent Results in Cancer Research
ISBN 978-3-319-42932-8 ISBN 978-3-319-42934-2 (eBook)
DOI 10.1007/978-3-319-42934-2

Library of Congress Control Number: 2016955320

Printed on acid-free paper

This Springer imprint is published by Springer Nature
The registered company is Springer International Publishing AG
The registered company address is: Gewerbestrasse 11, 6330 Cham, Switzerland

Contents

p53 Replacement Therapy for Cancer

Hiroshi Tazawa, Shunsuke Kagawa and Toshiyoshi Fujiwara

Abstract

Tumor suppressor gene (TSG) replacement therapy that involves various delivery systems is emerging as a promising antitumor strategy because malignant tumors develop through genetic alterations in TSGs. The most potent therapeutic TSG for tumor suppression is the multifunctional transcription factor p53 gene that regulates diverse cellular phenomena such as cell cycle arrest, senescence, apoptosis, and autophagy. Since the p53 gene is frequently inactivated by aberrant genetic regulation in human cancers, p53 replacement therapy is widely and frequently used as a potent antitumor strategy to restore wild-type p53 function in the p53-inactivated tumors. This chapter focuses on four types of p53 transfer systems: cationic liposome–DNA plasmid complexes, a replication-deficient adenovirus vector, a replication-competent adenovirus vector, and a protein transduction system. Moreover, we discuss recent advances in our understanding of the molecular basis of the p53-mediated cell death signaling pathway and therapeutic methods for enhancing tumor cell death and induction of bystander effects within tumor tissues in p53 replacement therapy. Exploration of the molecular mechanism underlying the p53-mediated tumor-suppressive network system and development of an effective strategy for enhancing p53-mediated cell death signaling pathways would lead to an improvement in the clinical outcome of patients with p53-inactivated cancers.

H. Tazawa
Center for Innovative Clinical Medicine, Okayama University Hospital, Okayama 700-8558, Japan

H. Tazawa · S. Kagawa · T. Fujiwara (✉)
Department of Gastroenterological Surgery, Okayama University Graduate School of Medicine, Dentistry and Pharmaceutical Sciences, 2-5-1 Shikata-cho, Okayama 700-8558, Japan
e-mail: toshi_f@md.okayama-u.ac.jp

W. Walther (ed.), *Current Strategies in Cancer Gene Therapy*,
Recent Results in Cancer Research 209, DOI 10.1007/978-3-319-42934-2_1

Keywords
Cancer · p53 · Gene therapy · Adenovirus

Abbreviations

TSG	Tumor suppressor gene
MDM2	Mouse double minute 2
DRAM	Damage-regulated autophagy modulator
hTERT	human telomerase reverse transcriptase
CAR	Coxsackie and adenovirus receptors
DCs	Dendritic cells

1 Introduction

Tumor suppressor gene (TSG) replacement therapy is emerging as a promising antitumor treatment for inducing programmed cell death via introduction of a therapeutic TSG (Roth and Cristiano 1997). Among the therapeutic TSGs for inducing tumor suppression, the most potent TSG is the p53 gene that functions as a multifunctional transcription factor for the regulation of diverse cellular phenomena such as cell cycle arrest, senescence, apoptosis, and autophagy (Vousden and Prives 2009). The IARC TP53 database (http://www-p53.iarc.fr/) (Olivier et al. 2002) indicates that various types of malignant tumors possess somatic mutations in the p53 gene (Olivier et al. 2010; Ognjanovic et al. 2012). The p53 gene is frequently inactivated by aberrant genetic regulation in human cancers, suggesting that the p53 gene plays a critical role in the tumor-suppressive network. Therefore, restoration of wild-type p53 function would be a promising antitumor strategy to strongly suppress the growth of p53-inactivated tumors.

p53 replacement therapy is widely and frequently used as a potent antitumor strategy to induce the expression of the p53 gene and subsequent cell death of many types of malignant tumors with p53-inactivated states (Roth et al. 1999; Fang and Roth 2003). To induce ectopic expression of an exogenous p53 gene or p53 protein, there are four types of p53 transfer systems: cationic liposome–DNA plasmid complexes, a replication-deficient adenovirus vector, a replication-competent adenovirus vector, and a protein transduction method. Activation of exogenous p53 expression efficiently induces p53-mediated cell death signaling pathways in the p53-inactivated tumor cells. In contrast, reactivation of endogenous p53 expression by treatment with chemical compounds such as Nutlin-3 (Selivanova 2014) or PRIMA-1 (Bykov and Wiman 2014) is another type of strategy to restore wild-type p53 function. Nutlin-3 induces p53 stabilization in tumor cells that overexpress p53-suppressive mouse double minute 2 (MDM2) through the inhibition of MDM2–p53 interaction (Vassilev et al. 2004). PRIMA-1 induces apoptosis by restoring DNA-binding activity and a functional conformation to a mutant p53 protein in human cancer cells with p53 gene mutation (Bykov et al. 2002). However, since the therapeutic potentials of Nutlin-3 and PRIMA-1 are limited to tumors with MDM2 overexpression and specific p53 gene mutations (R175H and R273H), respectively, p53 transfer systems for inducing exogenous p53 expression would provide useful antitumor strategies that could be more widely and frequently used in p53 replacement therapy.

This chapter focuses on the recent advances in p53 replacement therapy for the induction of overexpression of an exogenous p53 gene or p53 protein by using one of four types of p53 transfer systems: liposome-based p53 DNA plasmid delivery, replication-deficient adenovirus-based p53 gene delivery, replication-competent adenovirus-based p53 gene delivery, and membrane-permeable peptide-based p53 protein delivery. Furthermore, we will discuss the recent advances in our understanding of the molecular basis of the p53-mediated cell death signaling pathways induced by adenovirus vector and the molecular mechanism underlying an effective combination strategy for enhancing p53-mediated cell death against tumor cells.

2 p53-Mediated Cell Survival and Cell Death Signaling Pathways

In general, there are several types of p53-mediated cell death signaling pathways, including senescence, apoptosis, and autophagy (Fig. 1). When tumor cells with intact p53 function are under genotoxic stress, p53 is activated to transcriptionally induce many kinds of p53-downstream target genes, such as $p21^{WAF1}$ (p21) (el-Deiry et al. 1993), BAX (Miyashita and Reed 1995), or damage-regulated autophagy modulator (DRAM) (Crighton et al. 2006). Under mild genotoxic stress, p53 mainly upregulates p21 expression for the induction of cell cycle arrest that allows for the repair of DNA damage and contributes to cell survival. However, persistent cell cycle arrest by p21 activation results in the induction of senescence-associated cell death rather than cell survival. In contrast, severe genotoxic stress induces higher accumulation of p53, which activates BAX- and DRAM-related signaling pathways that lead to apoptosis and autophagy, respectively, and results in the induction of cell death. However, when the p53-downstream target gene MDM2 (Barak et al. 1993), which is a negative regulator of p53 via the ubiquitin–proteasome pathway, is upregulated following p53 activation, MDM2 activation inhibits the p53-mediated signaling pathway as a p53-negative feedback loop. Thus, the p53-mediated cell survival and cell death pathways are strictly regulated by many kinds of p53-downstream target genes.

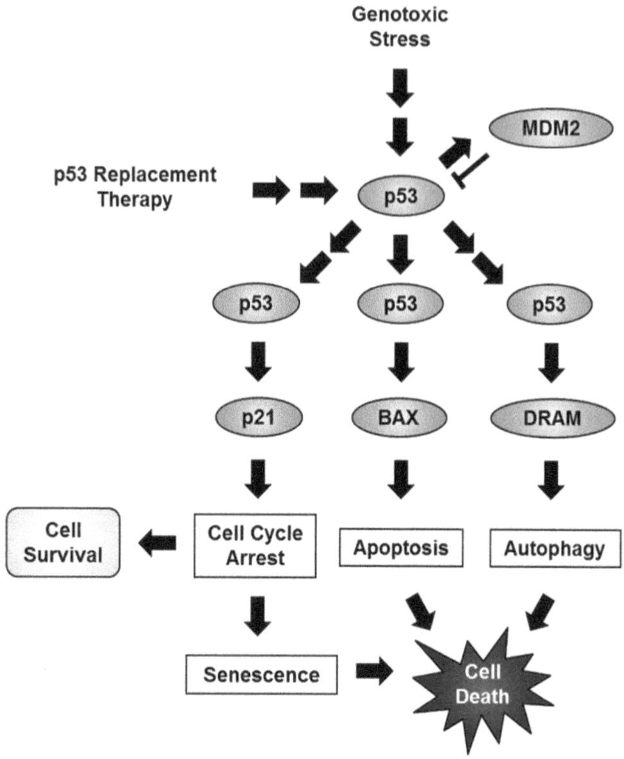

Fig. 1 Scheme of cell survival and cell death pathways induced by genotoxic stress or p53 replacement therapy. Genotoxic stress induces cell cycle arrest, apoptosis, or autophagy through the activation of the p53-target genes p21, BAX, or DRAM, respectively. Mild genotoxic stress induces accumulation of a small amount of p53, which contributes to p21-dependent cell cycle arrest and cell survival. However, severe genotoxic stress induces a large accumulation of p53, which results in the activation of three distinct cell death pathways: senescence, apoptosis, and autophagy. Moreover, p53-induced MDM2 activation functions as a p53-negative feedback loop via ubiquitin-mediated p53 degradation. In contrast, p53 replacement therapy induces p53-mediated cell death signaling pathways via the ectopic expression of exogenous p53 gene or p53 protein

3 p53 Replacement Therapy

To restore wild-type p53 function in a variety of p53-inactivated tumor cells, overexpression of an exogenous p53 gene or p53 protein by using one of several transfer methods is an effective strategy in preclinical and clinical settings (Fig. 1). Liposome-based p53 DNA plasmid delivery or virus-based p53 gene delivery transcriptionally activate ectopic expression of the exogenous p53 gene, whereas membrane-permeable peptide-based p53 protein delivery directly induces ectopic expression of the exogenous p53 protein. In the following sections, we demonstrate the therapeutic potential of p53 replacement therapy that involves a liposome–DNA plasmid complex, a replication-deficient virus vector, a replication-competent virus vector, or a protein transduction method, in preclinical and clinical settings.

3.1 Cationic Liposome Complex with a DNA Plasmid

Cationic liposomes are useful delivery systems for transfection of DNA plasmid vectors that encode ectopic p53 into human cancer cells in in vitro experiments (Xu et al. 1997; Zou et al. 1998; Ramesh et al. 2001; Nakase et al. 2005). To increase transfection efficiency and tumor-specific delivery of plasmid vectors, an antibody-conjugated immunoliposome has been recently developed for cancer treatment (Xu et al. 2001, 2002; Feng et al. 2009, 2010). However, transfection efficiencies using either liposome-based method are still low and are insufficient to induce cell death especially in in vivo tumor tissues. Therefore, improvement of liposome-based delivery systems is needed to efficiently induce p53-mediated cell death within tumor tissues.

3.2 Replication-deficient Adenovirus Vector

Compared to the low transfection efficiency of exogenous p53 induction with a plasmid DNA vector, a replication-deficient adenovirus Ad-p53 vector has been shown to efficiently induce expression of an exogenous p53 gene and exert a subsequent antitumor effect in preclinical in vitro and in vivo experiments (Fig. 2) (Roth et al. 1999; Fang and Roth 2003). The Ad-p53-mediated tumor-suppressive system includes three cell death pathways: senescence, apoptosis, and autophagy (Vousden and Prives 2009). These cell death pathways are determined by the induction of several p53-downstream target genes, such as p21 (el-Deiry et al. 1993), BAX (Miyashita and Reed 1995), or DRAM (Crighton et al. 2006) (Fig. 3).

To further promote Ad-p53-mediated cell death pathways, there are some combination strategies for enhancing viral replication, p53 expression, and p53-mediated cell death in the Ad-p53-infected tumor cells (Fig. 3). The first strategy is to use an E1A-expressing oncolytic adenovirus in combination therapy because Ad-p53 is an E1A-deleted replication-deficient adenovirus vector. For example, we previously generated a telomerase-specific replication-competent oncolytic adenovirus OBP-301 (Telomelysin) that induces tumor-selective cell lysis in a telomerase-dependent manner (Fig. 2) (Kawashima et al. 2004; Fujiwara et al. 2007; Hashimoto et al. 2008). OBP-301 enhanced Ad-p53-induced p53 expression in combination therapy, which resulted in a stronger antitumor effect and enhanced apoptotic cell death when compared to monotherapy with Ad-p53 (Sakai et al. 2010). Adenoviral E1A accumulation induced by OBP-301 was used for the replication of Ad-p53, which enhances Ad-p53-mediated p53 expression. A second strategy is to suppress MDM2 expression because p53-downstream activation of MDM2 inhibits p53 function via ubiquitin-mediated p53 degradation. Treatment with the small-molecule

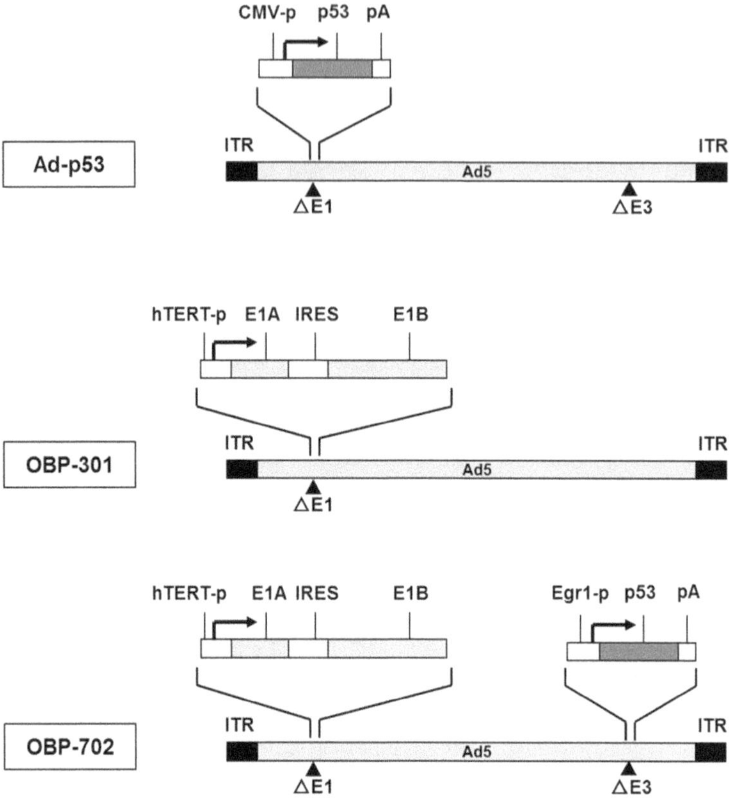

Fig. 2 DNA structures of Ad-p53, OBP-301, and OBP-702 vectors. The Ad-p53 vector is a p53-expressing replication-deficient adenovirus; a *p53* gene expression cassette that is under the regulation of the cytomegalovirus promoter (CMV-p) is inserted into the El region; the E3 region is deleted. The OBP-301 vector is a telomerase-specific replication-competent oncolytic adenovirus; the *hTERT* gene promoter (hTERT-p) element drives the expression of two adenoviral *E1A* and *E1B* genes that are linked to an internal ribosome entry site (IRES). The OBP-702 vector is a p53-expressing conditionally replicating adenovirus. In OBP-702, the p53 gene cassette controlled by the Egrl promoter (Egrl-p) is inserted into the E3 region of OBP-301

compound, Nutlin-3 (Graat et al. 2007), or infection with the tumor suppressor fragile histidine triad (*FHIT*) gene (Nishizaki et al. 2001) enhances Ad-p53-mediated p53 expression and apoptotic cell death through MDM2 suppression in human cancer cells. Furthermore, overexpression of the *ARF* gene by infection with Ad-ARF (Tango et al. 2002) or Ad-E2F1 (Itoshima et al. 2000) enhances p53 expression and the antitumor effect induced by Ad-p53 through ARF-mediated MDM2 suppression. A third strategy is to suppress p21 expression because p53-downstream p21 activation induces cell cycle arrest and subsequent cell survival. Suppression of p21 expression by genetic deletion (Gorospe et al. 1997) or an exogenous p21-targeted siRNA (Idogawa et al. 2009) enhances Ad-p53-induced apoptosis. Furthermore,

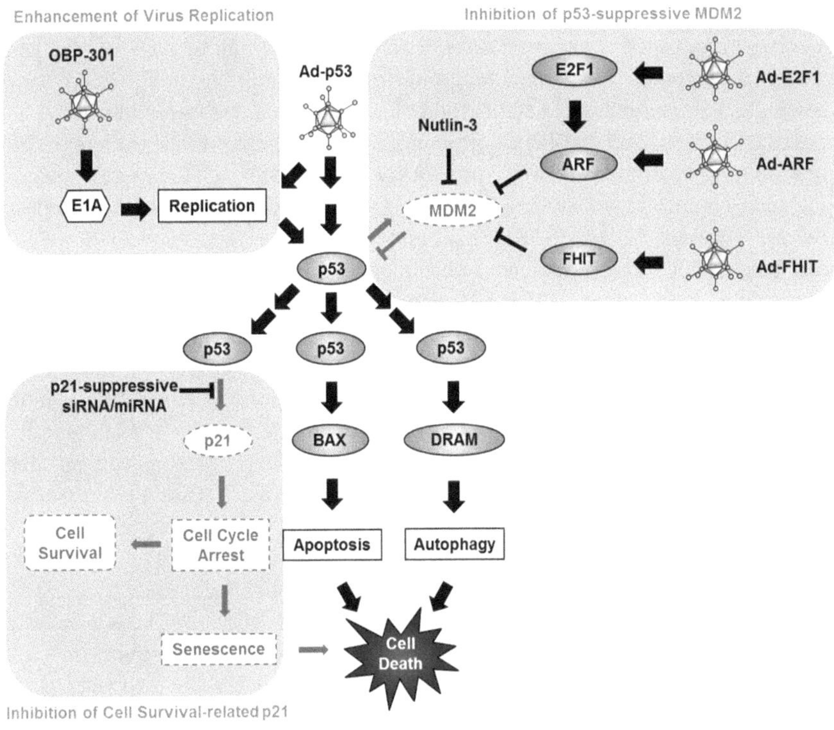

Fig. 3 A scheme for Ad-p53-mediated induction of cell death pathways and enhancement of Ad-p53-based p53 replacement therapy. The Ad-p53 vector induces BAX- and DRAM-mediated apoptosis and autophagy, respectively, resulting in cell death, rather than in p21-dependent cell cycle arrest and cell survival, when combined with E1A-expressing replication-competent OBP-301, several replication-deficient adenovirus vectors (Ad-E2F1, Ad-ARF, Ad-FHIT), Nutlin-3, or p21-suppressive siRNA/miRNA

p21-targeting miRNAs, *miR-93* and *miR-106b*, can enhance Ad-p53-mediated apoptosis and autophagy (Hasei et al. 2013) because p21 functions as a suppressor of apoptosis (Gorospe et al. 1997) and autophagy (Fujiwara et al. 2008). Thus, these three strategies for enhancing the Ad-p53-mediated cell death pathway are useful for improving the therapeutic potential of Ad-p53-based p53 gene replacement therapy.

3.3 Replication-competent Adenovirus Vector

Although a replication-deficient Ad-p53 vector has been shown to be safe, feasible, and well tolerated in patients with various types of cancers in many clinical studies (Tazawa et al. 2013), it may be hard to induce high exogenous p53 expression in all tumor cells by treatment with Ad-p53 because it is a replication-deficient virus. Therefore, the low transduction rate of p53 gene transfer via this replication-deficient

Ad-p53 vector is a major problem for the improvement of clinical outcome in patients with advanced cancers. To improve the transduction efficacy of p53 gene replacement therapy, tumor-specific, replication-competent oncolytic adenoviruses are being developed as novel vectors for anticancer gene therapies. For example, the promoters of cancer-related genes are being used to regulate virus replication in a tumor-dependent manner. We previously developed a telomerase-specific replication-competent oncolytic adenovirus OBP-301, in which the human telomerase reverse transcriptase (hTERT) promoter drives the expression of two adenoviral genes, *E1A* and *E1B*, that are linked to an internal ribosome entry site (Fig. 2) (Kawashima et al. 2004). OBP-301 can induce tumor-specific cell lysis in a telomerase-dependent manner (Kawashima et al. 2004; Fujiwara et al. 2007; Hashimoto et al. 2008). A phase I clinical study of OBP-301 was well tolerated by patients with advanced solid tumors in the USA (Nemunaitis et al. 2010). When Ad-p53 was combined with OBP-301, p53 expression and the antitumor effect induced by Ad-p53 were enhanced (Sakai et al. 2010) (Fig. 3). Based on these evidences, we generated an armed OBP-301 variant (OBP-702) that expresses the wild-type p53 gene under the control of the Egr1 promoter (Fig. 2). OBP-702 suppressed the viability of both OBP-301-sensitive and OBP-301-resistant tumor cells more efficiently than Ad-p53 or OBP-301 in epithelial and mesenchymal types of malignant tumor cells (Yamasaki et al. 2012; Hasei et al. 2013). Ad-p53 and OBP-301 mainly induced apoptotic and autophagic cell death, respectively, whereas OBP-702 caused both apoptotic and autophagic cell death via exogenous p53 overexpression in tumor cells. These results suggest that OBP-702 induces both apoptotic and autophagic cell death via high p53 overexpression.

Regarding the molecular mechanism by which OBP-702 is superior to Ad-p53 in inducing cell death, we recently found that E1A-dependent enhancement of the p53-mediated cell death signaling pathway was involved in the potent OBP-702-induced antitumor effect (Fig. 4). When tumor cells were infected with a similar dose of Ad-p53 or OBP-702, OBP-702 induced a higher level of p53 expression than Ad-p53 (Yamasaki et al. 2012; Hasei et al. 2013). This higher p53 expression is due to viral replication of OBP-702 because Ad-p53 is a replication-deficient type of virus. However, in spite of their higher p53 expression, the expression levels of the p53-downstream targets p21 and MDM2 were lower in the OBP-702-infected tumor cells than in the Ad-p53-infected tumor cells (Yamasaki et al. 2012). This difference between the expression levels of p53 and those of the p53-downstream targets p21 and MDM2 was due to adenoviral E1A accumulation. E1A accumulation induced the upregulation of E2F1-inducible *miR-93* and *miR-106b*, which suppressed p21 expression and resulted in the enhancement of p53-mediated apoptosis and autophagy (Hasei et al. 2013). In contrast, E1A-mediated E2F1 upregulation results in the suppression of MDM2 expression via ARF activation. These evidences suggest that OBP-702 induces an antitumor effect more efficiently than Ad-p53, via E1A-dependent enhancement of p53-mediated cell death signaling pathways.

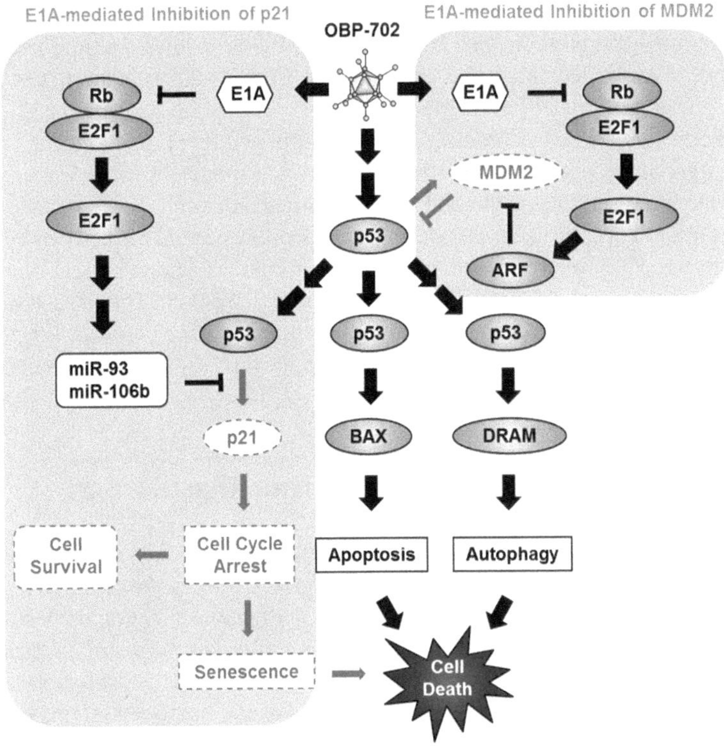

Fig. 4 Scheme for OBP-702-mediated induction of cell death pathways. The OBP-702 vector induces BAX- and DRAM-mediated apoptosis and autophagy, respectively, resulting in cell death; these effects are dependent on E1A-mediated suppression of p21 expression via E2F1-inducible miR-93 and miR-106b activation. Moreover, E1A-mediated suppression of MDM2, probably via E2F1-induced ARF activation, also enhances p53-mediated cell death

3.4 Protein Transduction Therapy

P53 replacement therapy using adenovirus vectors can induce ectopic expression of an exogenous p53 gene in various types of human cancers more strongly that induced by a plasmid-based delivery system. Since adenovirus can enter human cancer cells via direct interaction with virus particles and coxsackie and adenovirus receptors (CAR), CAR-expressing tumor cells are the main target cells for adenovirus-based p53 gene replacement therapy. However, CAR-negative tumor cells can escape from being eradicated by adenovirus-based p53 replacement therapy.

To target CAR-negative tumor cells, protein transduction therapy using membrane-permeable peptides may be useful for directly introducing exogenous p53 protein into tumor cells. For example, 11 polyarginine peptides fused to the p53 protein have been shown to introduce the p53 protein into cells, which subsequently induces the activity of the p21 gene promoter similar to the induction that occurs with Ad-p53-based p53 gene replacement therapy (Takenobu et al. 2002). Genetically modified p53 proteins that are resistant to MDM2-mediated ubiquitination are more effective in activating the transcription of p53-downstream target genes, resulting in a more potent antitumor effect compared to the wild-type p53 protein (Michiue et al. 2005). In contrast, introduction of wild-type p53 protein fused to three polyarginine peptides into cells cotreated with pyrenebutyrate was useful to induce the transcriptional activation of p53-downstream target genes (Hitsuda et al. 2012). Furthermore, by using this protein transduction system, the carboxy-terminal region of the p53 protein was shown to efficiently induce apoptosis and autophagy in human cancer cells (Li et al. 2005; Ueda et al. 2012). These accumulating evidences suggest that this protein transduction therapy using polyarginine peptides is a promising p53 replacement therapy especially for CAR-negative tumor cells.

4 Bystander Effect of p53 Replacement Therapy

P53 replacement therapy appears to induce cell death not only in p53-introduced tumor cells, but also in surrounding tumor cells through the activation of the bystander effect (Frank et al. 1998). The bystander effect is a biologic phenomenon in which non-treated tumor cells exhibit antitumor effects that are similar to those of treated tumor cells. In conventional antitumor therapy, a radiation-induced bystander effect is caused through the activation of the immune system, free radicals, and the inflammatory response (Najafi et al. 2014). In p53 replacement therapy, Ad-p53 treatment has been shown to induce a bystander effect on neighboring tumor cells through multiple mechanisms in preclinical in vivo situations (Fig. 5). For example, Ad-p53 infection decreased the expression of angiogenic factors including vascular endothelial growth factor and increased the expression of antiangiogenic factors, resulting in the suppression of angiogenesis within tumor tissues (Bouvet et al. 1998; Nishizaki et al. 1999). In contrast, activation of the immune response is also involved in the bystander effect induced by Ad-p53 (Fig. 5). Ad-p53 infection induced overexpression of the CD95 ligand, which caused both apoptosis via the Fas receptor/ligand system in infected tumor cells (Fukazawa et al. 1999) and massive infiltration of neutrophils within tumor tissues containing infected and non-infected tumor cells (Waku et al. 2000). When bone marrow-derived dendritic cells (DCs) were used as carrier cells for delivering Ad-p53, intratumoral injection with Ad-p53-integrated DCs caused an antitumor effect in both DC-injected and non-injected tumor tissues in subcutaneous xenograft tumor models (Murakami et al. 2004). Natural killer cells have been shown to be the immunologic mediators of the bystander effect induced by Ad-p53 (Carroll et al. 2001). These accumulating evidences suggest that p53 replacement therapy is a promising antitumor strategy for causing high cell death through the bystander effect-mediated modulation of the tumor microenvironment.

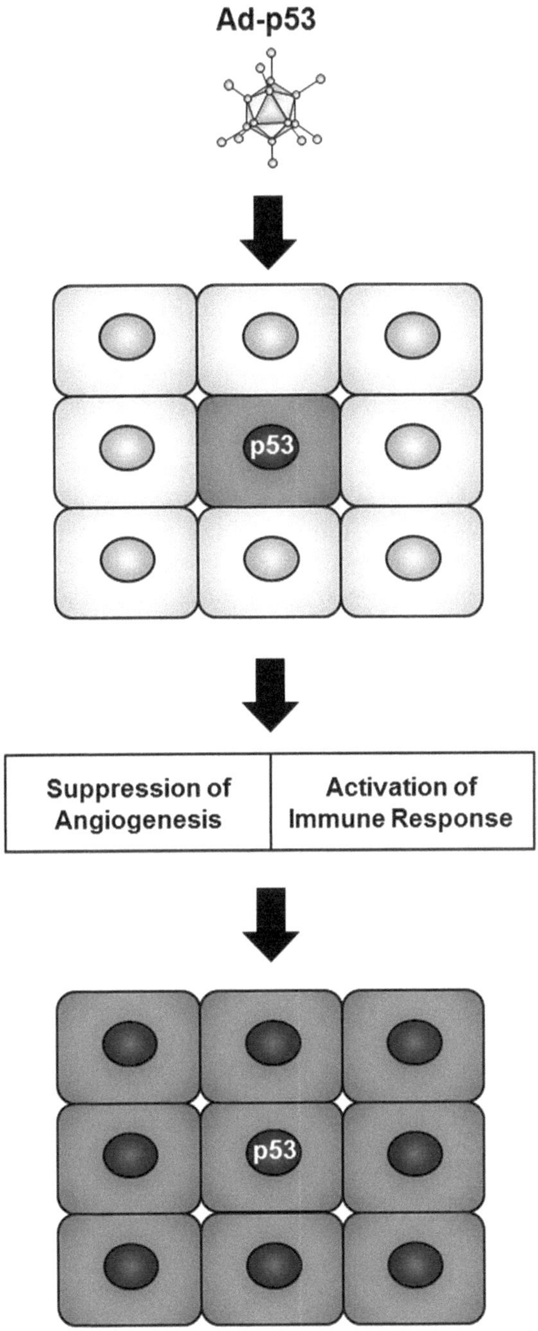

Fig. 5 A scheme for Ad-p53-mediated induction of bystander effects within tumor tissue. When tumor cells are infected with the Ad-p53 vector, ectopic expression of p53 induces programmed cell death in the Ad-p53-infected tumor cells. In addition, surrounding uninfected tumor cells are also eradicated via induction of bystander effects, which include suppression of angiogenesis and activation of immune responses, in the tumor microenvironment

5 Conclusion

P53 replacement therapy is emerging as a promising antitumor strategy for strong induction of p53-mediated cell death signaling pathways in tumor cells. Although a liposome-based delivery system is a useful method for in vitro experiments, the transduction efficiency is still lower than that of a virus-based delivery system in in vivo experiments. Many clinical studies using replication-deficient Ad-p53 vectors have demonstrated that administration of an Ad-p53 vector by one of several approaches, including intratumoral, intraperitoneal, and intravesical injection, is a safe, feasible, and effective antitumor strategy for patients with many types of cancers (Tazawa et al. 2013). However, although an Ad-p53 vector causes a bystander effect within tumor tissues, Ad-p53-mediated p53 activation may be insufficient for the induction of cell death in the entire tumor tissue because this virus is a replication-deficient virus. To improve the low transduction efficiency of adenovirus-based p53 replacement therapy, a replication-competent oncolytic adenovirus that expresses p53, OBP-702 (Yamasaki et al. 2012), has recently been developed (Fig. 2). In contrast, a protein transduction therapy using membrane-permeable polyarginine peptides would also be a useful strategy for introducing p53 into virus delivery-resistant tumor cells. Thus, given the underlying molecular mechanisms of p53-mediated cell death signaling pathways that are induced by various p53 transfer approaches, it should be possible to develop safer and effective p53 replacement therapy in the future.

Acknowledgments This study was supported by grants from the Ministry of Health, Labour, and Welfare of Japan and from the Ministry of Education, Culture, Sports, Science, and Technology of Japan.

References

Barak Y, Juven T, Haffner R, Oren M (1993) mdm2 expression is induced by wild type p53 activity. EMBO J 12(2):461–468

Bouvet M, Ellis LM, Nishizaki M, Fujiwara T, Liu W, Bucana CD, Fang B, Lee JJ, Roth JA (1998) Adenovirus-mediated wild-type p53 gene transfer down-regulates vascular endothelial growth factor expression and inhibits angiogenesis in human colon cancer. Cancer Res 58 (11):2288–2292

Bykov VJ, Wiman KG (2014) Mutant p53 reactivation by small molecules makes its way to the clinic. FEBS Lett 588(16):2622–2627

Bykov VJ, Issaeva N, Shilov A, Hultcrantz M, Pugacheva E, Chumakov P, Bergman J, Wiman KG, Selivanova G (2002) Restoration of the tumor suppressor function to mutant p53 by a low-molecular-weight compound. Nat Med 8(3):282–288

Carroll JL, Nielsen LL, Pruett SB, Mathis JM (2001) The role of natural killer cells in adenovirus-mediated p53 gene therapy. Mol Cancer Ther 1(1):49–60

Crighton D, Wilkinson S, O'Prey J, Syed N, Smith P, Harrison PR, Gasco M, Garrone O, Crook T, Ryan KM (2006) DRAM, a p53-induced modulator of autophagy, is critical for apoptosis. Cell 126(1):121–134 el-Deiry WS, Tokino T, Velculescu VE, Levy DB, Parsons R, Trent JM, Lin D, Mercer WE, Kinzler KW, Vogelstein B (1993) WAF1, a potential mediator of p53 tumor suppression. Cell 75(4):817–825

Fang B, Roth JA (2003) Tumor-suppressing gene therapy. Cancer Biol Ther 2(4 Suppl 1): S115–S121

Feng B, Tomizawa K, Michiue H, Miyatake S, Han XJ, Fujimura A, Seno M, Kirihata M, Matsui H (2009) Delivery of sodium borocaptate to glioma cells using immunoliposome conjugated with anti-EGFR antibodies by ZZ-His. Biomaterials 30(9):1746–1755

Feng B, Tomizawa K, Michiue H, Han XJ, Miyatake S, Matsui H (2010) Development of a bifunctional immunoliposome system for combined drug delivery and imaging in vivo. Biomaterials 31(14):4139–4145

Frank DK, Frederick MJ, Liu TJ, Clayman GL (1998) Bystander effect in the adenovirus-mediated wild-type p53 gene therapy model of human squamous cell carcinoma of the head and neck. Clin Cancer Res 4(10):2521–2528

Fujiwara T, Urata Y, Tanaka N (2007) Telomerase-specific oncolytic virotherapy for human cancer with the hTERT promoter. Curr Cancer Drug Targets 7(2):191–201

Fujiwara K, Daido S, Yamamoto A, Kobayashi R, Yokoyama T, Aoki H, Iwado E, Shinojima N, Kondo Y, Kondo S (2008) Pivotal role of the cyclin-dependent kinase inhibitor p21WAF1/CIP1 in apoptosis and autophagy. J Biol Chem 283(1):388–397

Fukazawa T, Fujiwara T, Morimoto Y, Shao J, Nishizaki M, Kadowaki Y, Hizuta A, Owen-Schaub LB, Roth JA, Tanaka N (1999) Differential involvement of the CD95 (Fas/APO-1) receptor/ligand system on apoptosis induced by the wild-type p53 gene transfer in human cancer cells. Oncogene 18(13):2189–2199

Gorospe M, Cirielli C, Wang X, Seth P, Capogrossi MC, Holbrook NJ (1997) p21(Waf1/Cip1) protects against p53-mediated apoptosis of human melanoma cells. Oncogene 14(8):929–935

Graat HC, Carette JE, Schagen FH, Vassilev LT, Gerritsen WR, Kaspers GJ, Wuisman PI, van Beusechem VW (2007) Enhanced tumor cell kill by combined treatment with a small-molecule antagonist of mouse double minute 2 and adenoviruses encoding p53. Mol Cancer Ther 6 (5):1552–1561

Hasei J, Sasaki T, Tazawa H, Osaki S, Yamakawa Y, Kunisada T, Yoshida A, Hashimoto Y, Onishi T, Uno F, Kagawa S, Urata Y, Ozaki T, Fujiwara T (2013) Dual programmed cell death pathways induced by p53 transactivation overcome resistance to oncolytic adenovirus in human osteosarcoma cells. Mol Cancer Ther 12(3):314–325

Hashimoto Y, Watanabe Y, Shirakiya Y, Uno F, Kagawa S, Kawamura H, Nagai K, Tanaka N, Kumon H, Urata Y, Fujiwara T (2008) Establishment of biological and pharmacokinetic assays of telomerase-specific replication-selective adenovirus. Cancer Sci 99(2):385–390

Hitsuda T, Michiue H, Kitamatsu M, Fujimura A, Wang F, Yamamoto T, Han XJ, Tazawa H, Uneda A, Ohmori I, Nishiki T, Tomizawa K, Matsui H (2012) A protein transduction method using oligo-arginine (3R) for the delivery of transcription factors into cell nuclei. Biomaterials 33(18):4665–4672

Idogawa M, Sasaki Y, Suzuki H, Mita H, Imai K, Shinomura Y, Tokino T (2009) A single recombinant adenovirus expressing p53 and p21-targeting artificial microRNAs efficiently induces apoptosis in human cancer cells. Clin Cancer Res 15(11):3725–3732

Itoshima T, Fujiwara T, Waku T, Shao J, Kataoka M, Yarbrough WG, Liu TJ, Roth JA, Tanaka N, Kodama M (2000) Induction of apoptosis in human esophageal cancer cells by sequential transfer of the wild-type p53 and E2F-1 genes: involvement of p53 accumulation via ARF-mediated MDM2 down-regulation. Clin Cancer Res 6(7):2851–2859

Kawashima T, Kagawa S, Kobayashi N, Shirakiya Y, Umeoka T, Teraishi F, Taki M, Kyo S, Tanaka N, Fujiwara T (2004) Telomerase-specific replication-selective virotherapy for human cancer. Clin Cancer Res 10(1 Pt 1):285–292

Li Y, Mao Y, Rosal RV, Dinnen RD, Williams AC, Brandt-Rauf PW, Fine RL (2005) Selective induction of apoptosis through the FADD/caspase-8 pathway by a p53 c-terminal peptide in human pre-malignant and malignant cells. Int J Cancer 115(1):55–64

Michiue H, Tomizawa K, Matsushita M, Tamiya T, Lu YF, Ichikawa T, Date I, Matsui H (2005) Ubiquitination-resistant p53 protein transduction therapy facilitates anti-cancer effect on the growth of human malignant glioma cells. FEBS Lett 579(18):3965–3969

Miyashita T, Reed JC (1995) Tumor suppressor p53 is a direct transcriptional activator of the human bax gene. Cell 80(2):293–299

Murakami T, Tokunaga N, Waku T, Gomi S, Kagawa S, Tanaka N, Fujiwara T (2004) Antitumor effect of intratumoral administration of bone marrow-derived dendritic cells transduced with wild-type p53 gene. Clin Cancer Res 10(11):3871–3880

Najafi M, Fardid R, Hadadi G, Fardid M (2014) The mechanisms of radiation-induced bystander effect. J Biomed Phys Eng 4(4):163–172

Nakase M, Inui M, Okumura K, Kamei T, Nakamura S, Tagawa T (2005) p53 gene therapy of human osteosarcoma using a transferrin-modified cationic liposome. Mol Cancer Ther 4 (4):625–631

Nemunaitis J, Tong AW, Nemunaitis M, Senzer N, Phadke AP, Bedell C, Adams N, Zhang YA, Maples PB, Chen S, Pappen B, Burke J, Ichimaru D, Urata Y, Fujiwara T (2010) A phase I study of telomerase-specific replication competent oncolytic adenovirus (telomelysin) for various solid tumors. Mol Ther 18(2):429–434

Nishizaki M, Fujiwara T, Tanida T, Hizuta A, Nishimori H, Tokino T, Nakamura Y, Bouvet M, Roth JA, Tanaka N (1999) Recombinant adenovirus expressing wild-type p53 is antiangiogenic: a proposed mechanism for bystander effect. Clin Cancer Res 5(5):1015–1023

Nishizaki M, Meyn RE, Levy LB, Atkinson EN, White RA, Roth JA, Ji L (2001) Synergistic inhibition of human lung cancer cell growth by adenovirus-mediated wild-type p53 gene transfer in combination with docetaxel and radiation therapeutics in vitro and in vivo. Clin Cancer Res 7(9):2887–2897

Ognjanovic S, Olivier M, Bergemann TL, Hainaut P (2012) Sarcomas in TP53 germline mutation carriers: a review of the IARC TP53 database. Cancer 118(5):1387–1396

Olivier M, Eeles R, Hollstein M, Khan MA, Harris CC, Hainaut P (2002) The IARC TP53 database: new online mutation analysis and recommendations to users. Hum Mutat 19(6): 607–614

Olivier M, Hollstein M, Hainaut P (2010) TP53 mutations in human cancers: origins, consequences, and clinical use. Cold Spring Harb Perspect Biol 2(1):a001008

Ramesh R, Saeki T, Templeton NS, Ji L, Stephens LC, Ito I, Wilson DR, Wu Z, Branch CD, Minna JD, Roth JA (2001) Successful treatment of primary and disseminated human lung cancers by systemic delivery of tumor suppressor genes using an improved liposome vector. Mol Ther 3(3):337–350

Roth JA, Cristiano RJ (1997) Gene therapy for cancer: what have we done and where are we going? J Natl Cancer Inst 89(1):21–39

Roth JA, Swisher SG, Meyn RE (1999) p53 tumor suppressor gene therapy for cancer. Oncology (Williston Park) 13(10 Suppl 5):148–154

Sakai R, Kagawa S, Yamasaki Y, Kojima T, Uno F, Hashimoto Y, Watanabe Y, Urata Y, Tanaka N, Fujiwara T (2010) Preclinical evaluation of differentially targeting dual virotherapy for human solid cancer. Mol Cancer Ther 9(6):1884–1893

Selivanova G (2014) Wild type p53 reactivation: from lab bench to clinic. FEBS Lett 588 (16):2628–2638

Takenobu T, Tomizawa K, Matsushita M, Li ST, Moriwaki A, Lu YF, Matsui H (2002) Development of p53 protein transduction therapy using membrane-permeable peptides and the application to oral cancer cells. Mol Cancer Ther 1(12):1043–1049

Tango Y, Fujiwara T, Itoshima T, Takata Y, Katsuda K, Uno F, Ohtani S, Tani T, Roth JA, Tanaka N (2002) Adenovirus-mediated p14ARF gene transfer cooperates with Ad5CMV-p53 to induce apoptosis in human cancer cells. Hum Gene Ther 13(11):1373–1382

Tazawa H, Kagawa S, Fujiwara T (2013) Advances in adenovirus-mediated p53 cancer gene therapy. Expert Opin Biol Ther 13(11):1569–1583

Ueda Y, Wei FY, Hide T, Michiue H, Takayama K, Kaitsuka T, Nakamura H, Makino K, Kuratsu J, Futaki S, Tomizawa K (2012) Induction of autophagic cell death of glioma-initiating cells by cell-penetrating D-isomer peptides consisting of Pas and the p53 C-terminus. Biomaterials 33(35):9061–9069

Vassilev LT, Vu BT, Graves B, Carvajal D, Podlaski F, Filipovic Z, Kong N, Kammlott U, Lukacs C, Klein C, Fotouhi N, Liu EA (2004) In vivo activation of the p53 pathway by small-molecule antagonists of MDM2. Science 303(5659):844–848

Vousden KH, Prives C (2009) Blinded by the light: the growing complexity of p53. Cell 137 (3):413–431

Waku T, Fujiwara T, Shao J, Itoshima T, Murakami T, Kataoka M, Gomi S, Roth JA, Tanaka N (2000) Contribution of CD95 ligand-induced neutrophil infiltration to the bystander effect in p53 gene therapy for human cancer. J Immunol 165(10):5884–5890

Xu L, Pirollo KF, Chang EH (1997) Transferrin-liposome-mediated p53 sensitization of squamous cell carcinoma of the head and neck to radiation in vitro. Hum Gene Ther 8(4):467–475. doi:10.1089/hum.1997.8.4-467

Xu L, Tang WH, Huang CC, Alexander W, Xiang LM, Pirollo KF, Rait A, Chang EH (2001) Systemic p53 gene therapy of cancer with immunolipoplexes targeted by anti-transferrin receptor scFv. Mol Med 7(10):723–734

Xu L, Huang CC, Huang W, Tang WH, Rait A, Yin YZ, Cruz I, Xiang LM, Pirollo KF, Chang EH (2002) Systemic tumor-targeted gene delivery by anti-transferrin receptor scFv-immunoliposomes. Mol Cancer Ther 1(5):337–346

Yamasaki Y, Tazawa H, Hashimoto Y, Kojima T, Kuroda S, Yano S, Yoshida R, Uno F, Mizuguchi H, Ohtsuru A, Urata Y, Kagawa S, Fujiwara T (2012) A novel apoptotic mechanism of genetically engineered adenovirus-mediated tumour-specific p53 overexpression through E1A-dependent p21 and MDM2 suppression. Eur J Cancer 48(14):2282–2291

Zou Y, Zong G, Ling YH, Hao MM, Lozano G, Hong WK, Perez-Soler R (1998) Effective treatment of early endobronchial cancer with regional administration of liposome-p53 complexes. J Natl Cancer Inst 90(15):1130–1137

Retroviral Vectors for Cancer Gene Therapy

Axel Schambach and Michael Morgan

Abstract

Advances in molecular technologies have led to the discovery of many disease-related genetic mutations as well as elucidation of aberrant gene and protein expression patterns in several human diseases, including cancer. This information has driven the development of novel therapeutic strategies, such as the utilization of small molecules to target specific cellular pathways and the use of retroviral vectors to retarget immune cells to recognize and eliminate tumor cells. Retroviral-mediated gene transfer has allowed efficient production of T cells engineered with chimeric antigen receptors (CARs), which have demonstrated marked success in the treatment of hematological malignancies. As a safety point, these modified cells can be outfitted with suicide genes. Customized gene editing tools, such as clustered regularly interspaced short palindromic repeats–CRISPR-associated nucleases (CRISPR-Cas9), zinc-finger nucleases (ZFNs), or TAL-effector nucleases (TALENs), may also be combined with retroviral delivery to specifically delete oncogenes, inactivate oncogenic signaling pathways, or deliver wild-type genes. Additionally, the feasibility of retroviral gene transfer strategies to protect the hematopoietic stem cells (HSC) from the

A. Schambach (✉) · M. Morgan (✉)
Institute of Experimental Hematology, Hannover Medical School, Hannover, Germany
e-mail: schambach.axel@mh-hannover.de

M. Morgan
e-mail: morgan.michael@mh-hannover.de

A. Schambach · M. Morgan
REBIRTH Cluster of Excellence, Hannover Medical School, Hannover, Germany

A. Schambach
Division of Hematology/Oncology, Boston Children's Hospital Harvard Medical School, Boston, MA, USA

W. Walther (ed.), *Current Strategies in Cancer Gene Therapy*,
Recent Results in Cancer Research 209, DOI 10.1007/978-3-319-42934-2_2

dose-limiting toxic effects of chemotherapy and radiotherapy was demonstrated. While some of these approaches have yet to be translated into clinical application, the potential implications for improved cellular replacement therapies to enhance and/or support the current treatment modalities are enormous.

Keywords
Retrovirus · Gene transfer · Anticancer · CAR · Gene editing · Cytoprotection

Abbreviations

aGVHD	Acute graft-versus-host disease
ALL	Acute lymphoblastic leukemia
AML	Acute myeloid leukemia
AraC	Cytarabine
CARs	Chimeric antigen receptors (CARs)
CLL	Chronic lymphocytic leukemia
CRISPR-Cas9	Clustered regularly interspaced short palindromic repeats–CRISPR-associated nucleases
CTLA-4	Cytotoxic T lymphocyte-associated antigen 4
DLBCL	Diffuse large-cell lymphoma
DNA	Deoxyribonucleic acid
EGFP	Enhanced green fluorescent protein
EGFR	Epidermal growth factor receptor
FL	Follicular lymphoma
HDR	Homology-directed repair
HLA	Human leukocyte antigen
HSC	Hematopoietic stem cells
HSPC	HSC and progenitor cells
HSV-tk	Herpes simplex virus thymidine kinase
IFN	Interferon
iPSC	Induced pluripotent stem cells
LTRs	Long-terminal repeats
MCL	Mantle cell lymphoma
MDR1	Multidrug resistance gene 1
MDS	Myelodysplastic syndrome
MGMT	O-6-methylguanine DNA methyltransferase
MPP	Multipotent progenitor
NB	Neuroblastoma
NHEJ	Nonhomologous end-joining
NSG	NOD.cgPrkdc^{scid}IL2rg$^{tm/Wjl}$/Sz
PD-1	Programmed death-1
preTs	T cell-committed progenitors
RD114/TR	Modified feline endogenous retrovirus envelope glycoprotein
RECIST	Response Evaluation Criteria in Solid Tumors

scFv	Single-chain variable fragment
SIN	Self-inactivating
TAA	Tumor-associated antigens
TALENs	TAL-effector nucleases
TCRs	T cell receptors
TERT	Telomerase
Thbd	Thrombomodulin
TNF	Tumor necrosis factor
ZFNs	Zinc-finger nucleases

1 Introduction

Curing cancer remains one of the greatest challenges facing the medical research and biotechnology fields. This task is complicated by the heterogeneity of cancer, with different tumor types exhibiting distinct genetic and phenotypic characteristics. For example, each acute myeloid leukemia (AML) genome is estimated to harbor approximately 13 coding mutations (Klco et al. 2014), while solid tumors of the colon, breast, brain, or pancreas contain 33–66 somatic mutations and melanomas and lung tumors have around 200 mutations (Vogelstein et al. 2013). The actual tumor burden of patients is often composed of different major and minor clones that may differ regarding capacity to engraft, proliferate, differentiate, transit from bone marrow to peripheral blood, and develop resistance (Klco et al. 2014). This makes the identification of the right target(s) critical for successful implementation of molecular-based therapies.

A key factor determining the clinical usefulness of any treatment modality is the successful delivery of the therapeutic agent. In the field of gene therapy, efficient transfer of the therapeutic gene technology to the target cell population is crucial. Retroviral vectors, including lentiviral vectors, are well known for their capacity to efficiently transduce a wide range of cell types and have been successfully used in the clinic (Aiuti et al. 2013; Biffi et al. 2013; Hacein-Bey-Abina et al. 2014; Naldini 2015) (Table 1). As the mechanism of action of retroviral vectors includes incorporation of the viral cargo into the target cell genome, therapies using retroviral vectors carry the risk of insertional mutagenic events in which viral insertion may deregulate the expression of proto-oncogenes or tumor suppressor genes. While some serious adverse events were observed in a subgroup of participants from the early gene therapy trials, these adverse events have not occurred in more recent trials using retroviral vectors with improved biosafety features, such as the use of self-inactivating (SIN) vectors in which viral promoters and enhancers have been deleted from the long-terminal repeats (LTRs), and transgene expression is driven by physiological promoters. Of note, the safety profile of any gene therapeutic

Table 1 Typical uses of retroviral vectors in human diseases in preclinical and clinical settings

Retrovirus	Cell target/topic	References
Foamy virus	HSC/WAS	Uchiyama et al. (2012)
Alpharetrovirus	HSC/X-CGD Pre T cells/leukemia T cells/GvHD NK cells/leukemia	Kaufmann et al. (2013) Hübner et al. (2016) Labenski et al. (2016) Suerth et al. (2016)
Gammaretrovirus	HSC/X-CGD HSC/ADA-SCID HSC/X-SCID (SIN vector) T cells/leukemia NK cells/gene transfer, neuroblastoma	Ott et al. (2006) Aiuti et al. (2002), Gaspar et al. (2011) Hacein-Bey-Abina et al. (2014) Brudno et al. (2016) Guven et al. (2005), Esser et al. (2012)
Lentivirus	HSC/ALD HSC/MLD HSC/WAS T cells/leukemia NK cells/gene transfer, glioblastoma	Cartier et al. (2009) Biffi et al. (2013) Aiuti et al. (2013) Kalos et al. (2011), Grupp et al. (2013), Maude et al. (2014), Porter et al. (2015) Micucci et al. (2006), Zhang et al. (2016)

Abbreviations HSC hematopoietic stem cell, *Pre T cells* precursor T cells, *NK cells* natural killer cells, *X-CGD* X-linked chronic granulomatous disease, *GvHD* graft-versus-host disease, *ADA-SCID* adenosine deaminase-deficient severe combined immunodeficiency, *X-SCID* X-linked severe combined immunodeficiency, *MLD* metachromatic leukodystrophy, *WAS* Wiskott–Aldrich syndrome

approach is also dependent upon the target cell population. For example, more primitive cells such as hematopoietic stem cells and precursor cells exhibit an inherently greater risk of transformation than differentiated cells such as T cells. Interestingly, even the use of gammaretroviral vectors with intact LTRs, which can be considered as one of the riskier retroviral vector configurations, for transduction of T cells has not resulted in any reported transformation events due to insertional mutagenesis (Newzeala et al. 2011, 2012; Heinrich et al. 2013).

Successful delivery and expression of therapeutic genes depend on several variables. For example, the retroviral vector system (i.e., the retroviral genus upon which the vector system is based) strongly influences the site of vector integration. Genomic analyses of murine and human HSC cells following transduction with alpharetroviral SIN vectors demonstrated a neutral genomic insertion site pattern and lower genotoxicity when compared to gammaretroviral or lentiviral SIN vectors (Suerth et al. 2012; Moiani et al. 2014). Gammaretroviral SIN vectors exhibited higher incidences of integrations near transcription start sites, CpG islands, and cancer-associated genes, while lentiviral SIN vectors preferentially integrated into actively transcribed genes. Importantly, retroviral gene delivery can be optimized for particular cell populations by choosing the viral envelope proteins compatible with the receptors expressed by the target cell population (Amirache et al. 2014). Additional factors that affect therapeutic gene transfer and expression in the target

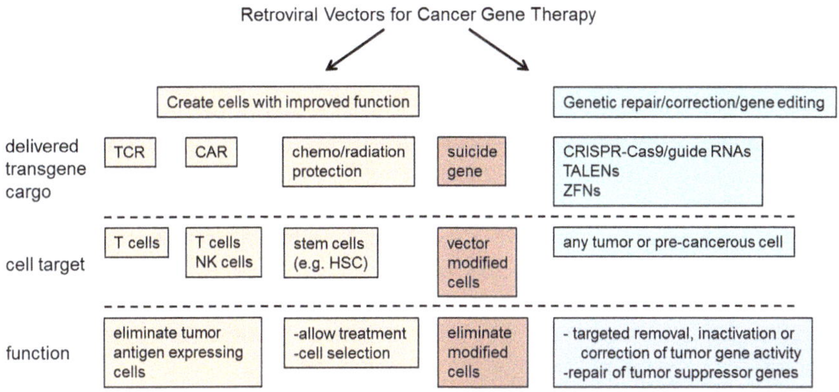

Fig. 1 Overview of retroviral vector use in cancer therapy. Retroviral vectors can be used to improve the immune cell antitumor activity or to protect the sensitive cell populations, such as HSC, from the cytotoxic effects of chemotherapy and radiotherapy (*orange boxes*). In addition to therapeutic genes, target cells can be cotransduced with suicide genes as a safety feature to eliminate the modified cells in case of undesirable effects, such as cell transformation or cytokine storm induction (*red boxes*). Gene editing techniques can be employed for the correction of tumor-specific genetic aberrations (*blue boxes*). *TCR* T cell receptor, *CAR* chimeric antigen receptor, *NK cells* natural killer cells, *HSC* hematopoietic stem cells, *CRISPR-Cas9* clustered regularly interspaced short palindromic repeats–CRISPR-associated nucleases, *TALENs* TAL-effector nucleases, *ZFNs* zinc-finger nucleases

cell include the strength and location of the promoter, transgene properties, the cell culture conditions, and the proliferative status of the cultured cells.

In this chapter, we discuss several available options to employ retroviral vectors in anticancer gene therapy treatment strategies, such as modification of immune cells with chimeric antigen receptors (CARs) or modified T cell receptors (TCRs), gene editing to inhibit oncogenic signals, and cell-protective and replacement approaches (Fig. 1).

2 Anticancer Strategies Based on CARs and TCR

Identification of tumor-associated antigens (TAA) has aided the development of monoclonal antibodies as cancer therapeutics (Scott et al. 2012). This strategy to target cancer cells was further exploited by engineering immune cells (e.g., T cells and NK cells) to express chimeric antigen receptors (CARs), which consist of an extracellular single-chain variable fragment (scFv) that recognizes a specific TAA. The scFv is coupled to intracellular costimulatory signaling domains (e.g., CD28, CD3ζ, 4-1BB, OX40, DAP10, and DAP12) that activate the cytotoxic function of the modified immune cell upon antigen recognition, resulting in specific elimination of cells expressing the TAA (e.g., the cancer cell) (Karlsson et al. 2015; Töpfer et al. 2015). Another strategy to create tumor-specific T cells is to use retroviral vectors to transfer T cell receptors (TCRs) engineered to exhibit improved binding affinity to a ligand specifically expressed on the target cancer cell population. T cell activation in response to antigen stimulation is modulated by costimulatory molecules, cell adhesion factors, and T cell receptor (TCR) affinity (van der Merwe and Davis 2003). Antigen recognition by CARs or TCRs directs T cell trafficking and accumulation in specific tissues, including tumors. TCRs can also be engineered to guide T cells to tumor tissue via the recognition of specific chemokines or components of the tumor microenvironment. For CAR- and TCR-based strategies, the targeted antigen should ideally be specifically expressed by tumor cells and not by healthy tissues, the antigen should induce an immunogenic response sufficient to eradicate the tumor, and the antigen should be important for the transformed phenotype, such as tumor cell survival, proliferation, metastasis, or resistance (Brentjens et al. 2013; Rapoport et al. 2015; Robbins et al. 2015; Sandri et al. 2016).

2.1 T Cells

Gammaretroviral and lentiviral vectors were used to generate T cells modified with CARs designed to target CD19, and these modified T cells (CART19, CTL019) were evaluated in clinical trials of pediatric and adult B cell malignancies (Kalos et al. 2011; Brentjens et al. 2013; Grupp et al. 2013; Maude et al. 2014; Porter et al. 2015; Brudno et al. 2016). In general, results from these trials were encouraging, with up to a 90 % (27/30 patients) complete response rate with a six-month overall survival rate of 78 % achieved in patients with relapsed or refractory acute lymphoblastic leukemia (ALL) (Maude et al. 2014). In chronic lymphocytic leukemia (CLL) patients, 57 % responded to CTL019 infusion and 29 % of patients achieved a long-lasting complete response (Porter et al. 2015). While CD19 is expressed on malignant B cells in several diseases, including chronic lymphocytic leukemia (CLL), acute lymphoblastic leukemia (ALL), diffuse large-cell lymphoma (DLBCL), follicular lymphoma (FL), and mantle cell lymphoma (MCL), it is also expressed on healthy B cells. Side effects due to CTL019 therapy include B cell aplasia, cytokine-release syndrome, tumor lysis syndrome, and neurological toxicities. The severity of these events varies in different disease settings, but most can be clinically managed (Namuduri and Brentjens 2016).

Successful disease control observed in trials using CD19-targeted T cells in patients with B-cell malignancies led to the development of CAR T cells for other cancers. Retroviral vectors were used to transfer an NY-ESO-1-specific TCR to T cells and tested in clinical trials for metastatic synovial cell sarcoma, melanoma, and myeloma (Robbins et al. 2015; Rapoport et al. 2015). The NY-ESO-1 antigen is expressed in 10–50 % of melanomas, 70–80 % of synovial cell sarcomas, and up to 60 % of advanced myelomas (Atanackovic et al. 2007; van Rhee et al. 2005). The absence of NY-ESO-1 expression on most adult human tissues makes this an interesting target for redirected T cell therapy. Objective clinical responses measured according to RECIST (Response Evaluation Criteria in Solid Tumors) guidelines were 61 % (11/18) in synovial cell sarcoma patients and 55 % (11/20) in melanoma patients (Robbins et al. 2015). Complete response or near-complete response was achieved in 70 % (14/20) of advanced multiple myeloma patients in a phase I/II trial testing lentiviral-mediated NY-ESO-1-specific TCR expression in T cells (Rapoport et al. 2015). NY-ESO-1-TCR expression was detected up to two years after modified T cell infusion, and loss of engineered T cells was associated with relapse (Rapoport et al. 2015).

It was recently demonstrated that T cells with an HLA-A2-restricted TCR modified to recognize telomerase (TERT) with high affinity successfully controlled human B-CLL progression in an in vivo murine model (Sandri et al. 2016). The main function of TERT is to maintain telomere ends. TERT expression is usually repressed in postnatal somatic cells, which contributes to senescence following a given number of cell divisions. TERT is often highly expressed in rapidly dividing cells such as embryonic stem cells, adult stem cells, and many types of tumor cells. Approximately 80–90 % of primary tumors exhibit high TERT expression, which is thought to contribute to the transformed phenotype. The "on-target, off-tumor" toxicity of TERT-directed T cells was mainly limited to mature granulocytes ($CD45^+CD11b^+CD16^+$), supporting further clinical development of this adoptive immunological anticancer strategy.

The antitumor efficacy of engineered T cells is at least partially a function of adequate expansion and engraftment of the modified cells. A preclinical trial in murine xenograft models of drug-resistant human ALL and CLL demonstrated that the combination of CAR T cell therapy with administration of the Bruton´s tyrosine kinase inhibitor ibrutinib improved CAR T cell engraftment and antileukemic activity (Fraietta et al. 2016). Analysis of $CD8^+$ T cells from CLL patients treated with five to eleven cycles of ibrutinib revealed decreased expression levels of the inhibitory receptor PD-1, suggesting that the reversal of T cell dysfunction also contributed to the enhanced antileukemic activity observed with this combination therapy (Fraietta et al. 2016).

2.2 T Precursor Cells

Retroviral vectors were used to transfer CARs or TCRs to T cell-committed progenitors (preTs) as a strategy to enhance the anticancer effects of preTs. While this approach eliminates the risk of graft-versus-host disease in allogeneic transplantation settings, it is important to use the safest retroviral vector design to limit the potential for serious adverse effects due to insertional mutagenesis, especially considering the inherent risk of transformation of precursor cell populations. A third-generation CAR engineered to target CD123-expressing cells was recently transferred to cord blood-derived $CD34^+$ cells, which were then differentiated in vitro into preTs (Hübner et al. 2016). SIN alpharetroviral vectors pseudotyped with a modified feline endogenous retrovirus envelope glycoprotein (RD114/TR) were used to obtain efficient transduction efficiency with minimized genotoxic risk. As an additional safety feature, the authors incorporated an inducible caspase 9 (iCasp9) cassette and demonstrated apoptosis of the modified cells upon introduction of the AP20187 dimerizing agent. CD123-CAR T cells produced IFNγ when cocultured with $CD123^+$ target cells and specifically lysed $CD123^+$ target cells. Importantly, CD123-CAR preTs engrafted into thymi of NSG (NOD. cgPrkdc^{scid}IL2rg$^{tm/Wjl}$/Sz) mice.

Transplantation of preTs engineered to inducibly express a leukemia-reactive TCR was recently shown to protect mice against repeated leukemia challenges via the generation of memory cells (Hoseini et al. 2015). The modified TCR was delivered via a lentiviral vector, and transduced preTs were enriched by sorting for the enhanced green fluorescent protein (EGFP) reporter. Interestingly, experiments investigating temporal control of TCR expression via doxycycline induction demonstrated that early induction of the modified TCR favored preT cell differentiation into $CD8^+$ T cells and allowed positive selection of the leukemia-reactive T cell subset (Hoseini et al. 2015).

2.3 NK Cells

Gammaretroviral- and lentiviral-mediated transfer of second-generation CARs into NK cell lines has been used to target neuroblastoma (NB) and glioblastoma tumors (Esser et al. 2012; Han et al. 2015; Zhang et al. 2016). GD2-expressing tumor cell lines and primary NB cells were selectively eliminated by GD2-specific-CAR-NK-92 clones in in vitro cocultivation experiments (Esser et al. 2012). The epidermal growth factor receptor (EGFR) is overexpressed in glioblastoma, but not in healthy brain tissue. Intracranial injection of NK-92 cells modified with an EGFR-CAR designed to target wild-type EGFR and the EGFRvIII mutant safely and efficiently eliminated EGFR-expressing glioblastoma tumor cells in an orthotopic xenograft model (Han et al. 2015). Elevated expression of ErbB2 (HER2), a growth factor receptor tyrosine kinase, was found in 41 % of primary glioblastomas and in several established glioblastoma cell lines (Zhang et al. 2016). NK-92 cells engineered via lentiviral gene transfer to express an ErbB2-CAR exhibited potent activity against glioblastoma cells in vitro and in in vivo orthotopic glioblastoma xenograft models (Zhang et al. 2016). These authors are planning a phase I clinical trial to test local application of ErbB2-CAR-NK-92 cells into the resection cavity in patients with recurrent ErbB2-positive glioblastoma.

T cells and NK cells engineered to express CARs may be used to support chemotherapy and radiotherapy treatment strategies to control or eliminate tumor cells. A systematic review combining patient outcome data from six phase I clinical trials testing CD-19 CAR T cells in refractory, relapsed, and advanced B cell malignancies showed that administration of conditioning chemotherapy was a statistically significant favorable factor in multivariate analysis for progression-free survival (Zhu et al. 2016). Increased T cell function, as measured by IFN-γ and TNF-α production, was observed in prostate cancer patients 24 h after a single low-dose pelvic radiation (Spary et al. 2014). In addition to reducing tumor burden, chemotherapy and radiotherapy may cause increased immunogenicity of tumor cells, thus allowing improved anticancer responses to CAR-modified immune cells.

2.4 Induced Pluripotent Stem Cells (iPSC)

Retroviral transfer of gene cassettes encoding the Yamanaka reprogramming transcription factors is well-established for the generation of induced pluripotent stem cells (iPSC), which exhibit a pluripotent embryonic stem cell-like phenotype (Takahashi and Yamanaka 2006). In principle, iPSC can be derived from any somatic cell type and possess the potential for differentiation into almost any type of tissue. These characteristics make iPSC interesting for disease modeling and regenerative medicine. For example, iPSC technology was used to model glioma tumor-initiating cells, which were then screened with a panel of small molecules to discover new potential treatment options and to improve our understanding of the mechanisms driving tumorigenesis (Sancho-Martinez et al. 2016). The feasibility of using iPSC technology to produce healthy hematopoietic cells devoid of leukemia-specific genetic alterations was recently demonstrated using either skin fibroblasts or bone marrow cells from AML patients (Salci et al. 2015; Hoffmann et al. 2016). These studies highlight the potential of iPSC technology to generate autologous, disease-free cell products for cellular replacement strategies.

3 Gene Therapy

Myelosuppression due to hematopoietic stem cell (HSC) sensitivity is a major dose-limiting toxicity for many chemotherapy and radiotherapy treatment approaches and may even cause interruption of scheduled therapy. One strategy to overcome this obstacle is to use retroviral gene transfer to confer protection to HSC or other desired cell populations. Exploitation of resistance mechanisms discovered in treatment refractory cancer cells, such as increased expression of enzymes important for DNA repair or expression of cellular efflux proteins that remove chemotherapeutic drugs from the cell, has driven the development of chemoresistant HSC.

3.1 O-6-Methylguanine DNA Methyltransferase (MGMT)

Introduction of genetically modified autologous HSC resistant to chemotherapy was used in glioblastoma patients to overcome treatment-related myelosuppression (Adair et al. 2012, 2014). One mechanism that tumor cells can become resistant to alkylating chemotherapies is through increased DNA repair activity. O-6-methylguanine DNA methyltransferase (MGMT) contributes to maintenance of genome stability via repair of the mutagenic DNA lesion O-6-methylguanine back to guanine (Tano et al. 1990). Intriguingly, decreased survival was observed in glioblastoma patients whose tumor cells lacked methylation of the promoter for the *MGMT* gene, presumably due to the increased MGMT expression and DNA repair activity in the tumor cells (Hegi et al. 2004). MGMT expression level was demonstrated to correspond to the extent of methylation in the *MGMT* gene promoter and coding region (Costello et al. 1994). Retroviral vector delivery of the $MGMT^{P140K}$ mutant protected primary murine bone marrow cells from alkylating agents (Moritz et al. 1995; Maze et al. 1999; Schambach et al. 2006). This therapeutic concept was translated into improved survival in glioblastoma patients (Adair et al. 2012, 2014). $MGMT^{P140K}$ modified HSC exhibited polyclonal engraftment and patients receiving these modified cells tolerated significantly more cycles of temozolomide/O-6-benzylguanine therapy.

3.2 Cytidine Deaminase and the Multidrug Resistance Gene 1 (MDR1)

Myelosuppression is also commonly observed in cancer patients treated with nucleoside analogs such as cytarabine (AraC), gemcitabine, azacytidine, and decitabine. Leukemia cells from patients with refractory acute myeloid leukemia (AML) were found to have elevated activity of cytidine deaminase, an enzyme involved in pyrimidine salvage and that catalyzes hydrolytic deamination of cytidine (Schröder et al. 1998). Increased cytidine deaminase expression and activity in male MDS and AML patients contributed to worse outcome as compared to females treated with azacytidine or decitabine (Mahfouz et al. 2013). Cytidine deaminase inhibitors, such as zebularine, can be used to overcome the tumor cell resistance to clinically used nucleoside analogs (Laliberté et al. 1992). Transfer of cytidine deaminase mutants resistant to zebularine may enhance the chemoprotection of HSC and thus reduce the life-threatening myelosuppression during nucleoside analog treatment (Ruan et al. 2016). Standard cytotoxic chemotherapy for high-risk myelodysplastic syndrome (MDS) and AML consists of a combination of AraC and anthracycline administration (Büchner et al. 2012). P-glycoprotein, a cellular efflux protein coded for by the *MDR1* gene, confers resistance to anthracyclines and other chemotherapeutic agents (Shen et al. 1986). Concomitant lentiviral-mediated gene transfer of cytidine deaminase and the multidrug resistance gene 1 (*MDR1*) protected primary murine hematopoietic stem and progenitor cells from AraC and anthracycline treatment (Brennig et al. 2015).

Lentiviral vector delivery of *MDR1* was also shown to protect human $CD34^+$ HSC and progenitor cells (HSPC) against radiation-induced toxicity (Maier et al. 2008). The mechanism of radioprotection by elevated *MDR1* expression remains to be demonstrated, but may involve upregulation of detoxifying proteins and inhibition of apoptosis by suppression of caspase activity (Maier et al. 2006). A retroviral insertional mutagenesis screen to identify pathways that protect HSPC from irradiation found retroviral vector insertion upstream of thrombomodulin

(*Thbd*), which resulted in elevated *Thbd* expression in radiation-selected cells (Geiger et al. 2012). Lentiviral-mediated thrombomodulin ectopic expression in murine HSPC or endothelial and stromal cells from the bone marrow compartment protected HSPC as demonstrated by an in vivo selection advantage following irradiation (Geiger et al. 2012). Another viral vector integration site discovered in this study was in the gene locus of *Puma*. PUMA mediates p53-induced apoptosis in HSPC and hematopoietic multipotent progenitors (MPP), and repression of PUMA was demonstrated to be important for MPP survival and maintenance of the HSC pool (Belle et al. 2016). Thus, the use of retroviral vectors designed to express cell-protective genes or to downregulate the expression of cell-destructive genes may be useful to combat toxicity to healthy cell compartments.

3.3 Suicide Gene Strategies

The use of retroviral strategies may require some alternative means for removal of the transduced cell populations in the event of an undesired cell transformation event. Several options for this eventuality have been created, including incorporation of suicide genes into the retroviral gene cassette transferred to the therapeutic cells. Herpes simplex virus thymidine kinase (HSV-tk) kills dividing cells by mediating conversion of ganciclovir to the cytotoxic ganciclovir triphosphate. HSV-tk-modified T cells were efficiently eradicated by ganciclovir administration, thus resolving acute graft-versus-host disease (aGVHD) in a clinical trial designed to test this strategy for improved allogeneic bone marrow transplantation safety and efficacy (Bonini et al. 1997). Since HSV-tk is a foreign protein, strategies employing HSV-tk may induce immunogenicity leading to purging of the modified cells earlier than desired (Berger et al. 2006). Another potential challenge is outgrowth of ganciclovir-resistant clones due to silencing of *HSV-tk* gene expression in modified cells (Frank et al. 2004). Additional strategies to remove gene-modified cells in the case of severe adverse events include the use of apoptosis-inducing fusion proteins (e.g., inducible Fas or Caspase 9) or expression of cell surface markers compatible with antibodies for cell depletion (e.g., CD20 can be depleted with rituximab, and truncated epidermal growth factor receptor can be depleted with cetuximab) (Straathof et al. 2005; Vogler et al. 2010; Wang et al. 2011).

3.4 Genome Editing Strategies

Recent advances in molecular biological technologies make specific directed genome editing possible. In principle, after the identification of the genetic lesion causative for tumor cell survival and propagation, techniques employing nucleases such as CRISPR-Cas9, ZFNs, or TALENs can be employed to excise, correct, or silence the respective oncogene(s). DNA double-strand breaks generated by nucleases can be repaired by nonhomologous end-joining (NHEJ) or homology-directed repair (HDR). Insertion and deletion mutations can be generated by NHEJ and may disrupt gene transcription or translation. Point mutations can be corrected via a dead Cas9 fused to a cytidine deaminase enzyme (Komor et al. 2016). The CRISPR-Cas9 genetic engineering system is based on a bacterial innate immune system, and the genetic editing site can be programmed using an RNA guide sequence to direct cleavage to a specific DNA sequence (Jinek et al. 2012). ZFN and TALEN approaches both use protein–DNA interactions to specifically cleave the genomic DNA at a desired locus.

Retroviral vector technology can be used to deliver CRISPR-Cas9, ZFNs, or TALENs to cancer cells. Lentiviral delivery of a CRISPR-Cas9 knockout library to human melanoma cells was used to discover novel genes important for resistance to vemurafenib, a targeted therapy designed to inhibit activated BRAF mutants (Shalem et al. 2014). Lentivirus-derived particles were used for efficient delivery of ZFN and TALEN proteins into cell lines and primary human keratinocytes (Cai et al. 2014). Efficient delivery of TALENs as mRNA was demonstrated with lentiviral particles containing inactivated reverse transcriptase (Mock et al. 2014). These gene editing technologies can be designed to excise, silence, or correct specific oncogenes/genetic alterations relevant to human cancer. For example, TALEN-mediated disruption of *FLT3*, a commonly mutated gene in AML, was demonstrated in leukemia cell lines (Wang et al. 2015). Lentiviral delivery of CRISPR-Cas9 to mediate genome editing of tumor suppressor genes in an inducible $Kras^{G12D}$ murine lung tumor model allowed identification of cooperating genetic events, such as deletion of *Nkx2-1*, *Pten*, and *Apc* that may contribute to tumorigenesis and progression (Sánchez-Rivera et al. 2014). Genome editing technologies can be used to create disease models based on whole genome sequencing data that are available for many different types of cancers. Additionally, loss of function screening with CRISPR-Cas9 and genome-wide lentiviral guide RNA libraries can be used to create homozygous gene knockouts, which will help create improved disease models by overcoming the problem of incomplete suppression of gene expression common in RNA interference technologies (Koike-Yusa et al. 2014). Targeted gene correction or inactivation of tumor-specific genetic aberrations, including fusion proteins such as BCR-ABL, RUNX1-ETO, PML-RARA, and NPM-ALK, that are causative for cancer may one day be a possible treatment option.

4 Conclusions

Recent advances in available technology have led to greater understanding of the genetic aberrations that cause many types of cancer. Our current challenge is to use this information to design better treatment strategies to control or cure cancer. Retroviral vectors are efficient tools for cell modification, and several types of cells engineered with these vectors are used in clinical trials. Improved retroviral vector designs have increased the safety of gene transfer, and no vector-related serious adverse effects have occurred in any of the patients treated in clinical trials with the new SIN vector platform (Aiuti et al. 2013; Biffi et al. 2013; Hacein-Bey-Abina et al. 2014; Naldini 2015). As described above, retroviral gene transfer can be used to change cell fate, improve fitness (confer protection), alter proliferation, and to change cell behavior. Development of stable packaging cell lines might solve challenges, such as costs and efforts associated with scaling up viral vector production to meet the increased demand for GMP-grade retroviral vectors suitable for clinical use (Labenski et al. 2016).

The success of recent trials, in which effective control of B cell lymphomas by transfer of CAR-modified T cells was demonstrated, is a driving force behind the search for suitable targets in other hematological and solid cancers. Challenges such as tumor heterogeneity, where expression of the target antigen may be low or even absent on some tumor cells, may require reconsideration of current CAR strategies. For example, three ALL patients who initially responded to CD19 CAR T cell therapy relapsed with $CD19^{-}$ leukemia (Singh et al. 2016). Thus, it might be necessary to generate and deliver immune cells modified to detect more than a single TAA to treat some cancers. Infusion of a pool of immune cells targeting a limited number of TAAs is expected to produce improved disease control, but must be carefully tested to limit the undesired toxicity to healthy tissue. Therapeutic regimens incorporating redirected immune cells may allow improved disease control with decreased doses of chemo- and/or radiotherapies, thus limiting non-specific toxicities. Dose-limiting toxicities, such as suppression of the hematopoietic compartment, associated with chemotherapies and irradiation strategies may also be overcome by the protection of HSC and progenitors with gene therapy.

Effectiveness of T cell therapies can be limited by immunosuppressive pathways, such as expression of the inhibitory immune receptors cytotoxic T lymphocyte-associated antigen 4 (CTLA-4) or programmed death-1 (PD-1) after T cell activation (Pardoll 2012). CAR T cell therapy was improved in a Her-2 transgenic murine breast cancer model by dual treatment with anti-Her-2 T cells and an anti-PD-1 antibody (John et al. 2013). Treatment modalities combining CAR T cells with checkpoint inhibitors designed to target PD-1 and CTLA-4 may be more effective, but the potential adverse events must be carefully monitored.

The use of retroviral gene therapy to deliver genome editing tools represents a major technological advancement that combines efficient gene transfer with the potential for site-specific genetic modification. If we can safely harness the immense power of these molecular tools, cell and gene-specific therapies will become a reality, allowing improved treatment and possibly eradication of many cancers.

Acknowledgments This work was supported by grants from the Deutsche Forschungsgemeinschaft [SFB738, Cluster of Excellence REBIRTH (EXC 62/1)], the Bundesministerium für Bildung und Forschung (BMBF, Joint Research Project IFB-Tx, PID-NET), CRISPR Therapeutics and the European Union (FP7 projects PERSIST, CELLPID and Horizon 2020 project SCIDNET).

References

Adair JE, Beard BC, Trobridge GD, Neff T, Rockhill JK, Silbergeld DL, Mrugala MM, Kiem HP (2012) Extended survival of glioblastoma patients after chemoprotective HSC gene therapy. Sci Transl Med 4(133):133ra57

Adair JE, Johnston SK, Mrugala MM, Beard BC, Guyman LA, Baldock AL, Bridge CA, Hawkins-Daarud A, Gori JL, Born DE, Gonzalez-Cuyar LF, Silbergeld DL, Rockne RC, Storer BE, Rockhill JK, Swanson KR, Kiem HP (2014) Gene therapy enhances chemotherapy tolerance and efficacy in glioblastoma patients. J Clin Invest 124(9):4082–4092

Aiuti A, Slavin S, Aker M, Ficara F, Deola S, Mortellaro A, Morecki S, Andolfi G, Tabucchi A, Carlucci F, Marinello E, Cattaneo F, Vai S, Servida P, Miniero R, Roncarolo MG, Bordignon C (2002) Correction of ADA-SCID by stem cell gene therapy combined with nonmyeloablative conditioning. Science 296(5577):2410–2413

Aiuti A, Biasco L, Scaramuzza S, Ferrua F, Cicalese MP, Baricordi C, Dionisio F, Calabria A, Giannelli S, Castiello MC, Bosticardo M, Evangelio C, Assanelli A, Casiraghi M, Di Nunzio S, Callegaro L, Benati C, Rizzardi P, Pellin D, Di Serio C, Schmidt M, Von Kalle C, Gardner J, Mehta N, Neduva V, Dow DJ, Galy A, Miniero R, Finocchi A, Metin A, Banerjee PP, Orange JS, Galimberti S, Valsecchi MG, Biffi A, Montini E, Villa A, Ciceri F, Roncarolo MG, Naldini L (2013) Lentiviral hematopoietic stem cell gene therapy in patients with Wiskott-Aldrich syndrome. Science 341(6148):1233151

Amirache F, Lévy C, Costa C, Mangeot PE, Torbett BE, Wang CX, Nègre D, Cosset FL, Verhoeyen E (2014) Mystery solved: VSV-G-LVs do not allow efficient gene transfer into unstimulated T cells, B cells, and HSCs because they lack the LDL receptor. Blood 123 (9):1422–1424

Atanackovic D, Arfsten J, Cao Y, Gnjatic S, Schnieders F, Bartels K, Schilling G, Faltz C, Wolschke C, Dierlamm J, Ritter G, Eiermann T, Hossfeld DK, Zander AR, Jungbluth AA, Old LJ, Bokemeyer C, Kröger N (2007) Cancer-testis antigens are commonly expressed in multiple myeloma and induce systemic immunity following allogeneic stem cell transplantation. Blood 109(3):1103–1112

Belle JI, Petrov JC, Langlais D, Robert F, Cencic R, Shen S, Pelletier J, Gros P, Nijnik A (2016) Repression of p53-target gene Bbc3/PUMA by MYSM1 is essential for the survival of hematopoietic multipotent progenitors and contributes to stem cell maintenance. Cell Death Differ 23(5):759–775

Berger C, Flowers ME, Warren EH, Riddell SR (2006) Analysis of transgene-specific immune responses that limit the in vivo persistence of adoptively transferred HSV-TK-modified donor T cells after allogeneic hematopoietic cell transplantation. Blood 107:2294–2302

Biffi A, Montini E, Lorioli L, Cesani M, Fumagalli F, Plati T, Baldoli C, Martino S, Calabria A, Canale S, Benedicenti F, Vallanti G, Biasco L, Leo S, Kabbara N, Zanetti G, Rizzo WB, Mehta NA, Cicalese MP, Casiraghi M, Boelens JJ, Del Carro U, Dow DJ, Schmidt M, Assanelli A, Neduva V, Di Serio C, Stupka E, Gardner J, von Kalle C, Bordignon C, Ciceri F, Rovelli A, Roncarolo MG, Aiuti A, Sessa M, Naldini L (2013) Lentiviral hematopoietic stem cell gene therapy benefits metachromatic leukodystrophy. Science 341(6148):1233158

Bonini C, Ferrari G, Verzeletti S, Servida P, Zappone E, Ruggieri L, Ponzoni M, Rossini S, Mavilio F, Traversari C, Bordignon C (1997) HSV-TK gene transfer into donor lymphocytes for control of allogeneic graft-versus-leukemia. Science 276(5319):1719–1724

Brennig S, Lachmann N, Buchegger T, Hetzel M, Schambach A, Moritz T (2015) Chemoprotection of murine hematopoietic cells by combined gene transfer of cytidine deaminase (CDD) and multidrug resistance 1 gene (MDR1). J Exp Clin Cancer Res 34:148

Brentjens RJ, Davila ML, Riviere I, Park J, Wang X, Cowell LG, Bartido S, Stefanski J, Taylor C, Olszewska M, Borquez-Ojeda O, Qu J, Wasielewska T, He Q, Bernal Y, Rijo IV, Hedvat C, Kobos R, Curran K, Steinherz P, Jurcic J, Rosenblat T, Maslak P, Frattini M, Sadelain M (2013) CD19-targeted T cells rapidly induce molecular remissions in adults with chemotherapy-refractory acute lymphoblastic leukemia. Sci Transl Med 5(177):177ra38

Brudno JN, Somerville RP, Shi V, Rose JJ, Halverson DC, Fowler DH, Gea-Banacloche JC, Pavletic SZ, Hickstein DD, Lu TL, Feldman SA, Iwamoto AT, Kurlander R, Maric I, Goy A, Hansen BG, Wilder JS, Blacklock-Schuver B, Hakim FT, Rosenberg SA, Gress RE, Kochenderfer JN (2016) Allogeneic T Cells that express an anti-CD19 chimeric antigen receptor induce remissions of B-Cell malignancies that progress after allogeneic hematopoietic stem-cell transplantation without causing graft-versus-host disease. J Clin Oncol 34(10):1112–1121

Büchner T, Schlenk RF, Schaich M, Döhner K, Krahl R, Krauter J, Heil G, Krug U, Sauerland MC, Heinecke A, Späth D, Kramer M, Scholl S, Berdel WE, Hiddemann W, Hoelzer D, Hehlmann R, Hasford J, Hoffmann VS, Döhner H, Ehninger G, Ganser A, Niederwieser DW, Pfirrmann M (2012) Acute Myeloid Leukemia (AML): different treatment strategies versus a common standard arm–combined prospective analysis by the German AML Intergroup. J Clin Oncol 30(29):3604–3610

Cai Y, Bak RO, Mikkelsen JG (2014) Targeted genome editing by lentiviral protein transduction of zinc-finger and TAL-effector nucleases. Elife 3:e01911

Cartier N, Hacein-Bey-Abina S, Bartholomae CC, Veres G, Schmidt M, Kutschera I, Vidaud M, Abel U, Dal-Cortivo L, Caccavelli L, Mahlaoui N, Kiermer V, Mittelstaedt D, Bellesme C, Lahlou N, Lefrère F, Blanche S, Audit M, Payen E, Leboulch P, l'Homme B, Bougnères P, Von Kalle C, Fischer A, Cavazzana-Calvo M, Aubourg P (2009) Hematopoietic stem cell gene therapy with a lentiviral vector in X-linked adrenoleukodystrophy. Science 326(5954):818–823

Costello JF, Futscher BW, Tano K, Graunke DM, Pieper RO (1994) Graded methylation in the promoter and body of the O6-methylguanine DNA methyltransferase (MGMT) gene correlates with MGMT expression in human glioma cells. J Biol Chem 269(25):17228–17237

Esser R, Müller T, Stefes D, Kloess S, Seidel D, Gillies SD, Aperlo-Iffland C, Huston JS, Uherek C, Schönfeld K, Tonn T, Huebener N, Lode HN, Koehl U, Wels WS (2012) NK cells engineered to express a GD2-specific antigen receptor display built-in ADCC-like activity against tumour cells of neuroectodermal origin. J Cell Mol Med 16(3):569–581

Fraietta JA, Beckwith KA, Patel PR, Ruella M, Zheng Z, Barrett DM, Lacey SF, Melenhorst JJ, McGettigan SE, Cook DR, Zhang C, Xu J, Do P, Hulitt J, Kudchodkar SB, Cogdill AP, Gill S, Porter DL, Woyach JA, Long M, Johnson AJ, Maddocks K, Muthusamy N, Levine BL, June CH, Byrd JC, Maus MV (2016) Ibrutinib enhances chimeric antigen receptor T-cell engraftment and efficacy in leukemia. Blood 127(9):1117–1127

Frank O, Rudolph C, Heberlein C, von Neuhoff N, Schrock E, Schambach A, Schlegelberger B, Fehse B, Ostertag W, Stocking C, Baum C (2004) Tumor cells escape suicide gene therapy by genetic and epigenetic instability. Blood 104:3543–3549

Gaspar HB, Cooray S, Gilmour KC, Parsley KL, Zhang F, Adams S, Bjorkegren E, Bayford J, Brown L, Davies EG, Veys P, Fairbanks L, Bordon V, Petropoulou T, Kinnon C, Thrasher AJ (2011) Hematopoietic stem cell gene therapy for adenosine deaminase-deficient severe combined immunodeficiency leads to long-term immunological recovery and metabolic correction. Sci Transl Med 3(97):97ra80

Geiger H, Pawar SA, Kerschen EJ, Nattamai KJ, Hernandez I, Liang HP, Fernández JÁ, Cancelas JA, Ryan MA, Kustikova O, Schambach A, Fu Q, Wang J, Fink LM, Petersen KU, Zhou D, Griffin JH, Baum C, Weiler H, Hauer-Jensen M (2012) Pharmacological targeting of the thrombomodulin-activated protein C pathway mitigates radiation toxicity. Nat Med 18 (7):1123–1129

Grupp SA, Kalos M, Barrett D, Aplenc R, Porter DL, Rheingold SR, Teachey DT, Chew A, Hauck B, Wright JF, Milone MC, Levine BL, June CH (2013) Chimeric antigen receptor-modified T cells for acute lymphoid leukemia. N Engl J Med 368(16):1509–1518

Guven H, Konstantinidis KV, Alici E, Aints A, Abedi-Valugerdi M, Christensson B, Ljunggren HG, Dilber MS (2005) Efficient gene transfer into primary human natural killer cells by retroviral transduction. Exp Hematol 33:1320–1328

Hacein-Bey-Abina S, Pai SY, Gaspar HB, Armant M, Berry CC, Blanche S, Bleesing J, Blondeau J, de Boer H, Buckland KF, Caccavelli L, Cros G, De Oliveira S, Fernández KS, Guo D, Harris CE, Hopkins G, Lehmann LE, Lim A, London WB, van der Loo JC, Malani N,

Male F, Malik P, Marinovic MA, McNicol AM, Moshous D, Neven B, Oleastro M, Picard C, Ritz J, Rivat C, Schambach A, Shaw KL, Sherman EA, Silberstein LE, Six E, Touzot F, Tsytsykova A, Xu-Bayford J, Baum C, Bushman FD, Fischer A, Kohn DB, Filipovich AH, Notarangelo LD, Cavazzana M, Williams DA, Thrasher AJ (2014) A modified γ-retrovirus vector for X-linked severe combined immunodeficiency. N Engl J Med 371(15):1407–1417

Han J, Chu J, Keung Chan W, Zhang J, Wang Y, Cohen JB, Victor A, Meisen WH, Kim SH, Grandi P, Wang QE, He X, Nakano I, Chiocca EA, Glorioso JC 3rd, Kaur B, Caligiuri MA, Yu J (2015) CAR-engineered NK cells targeting wild-type EGFR and EGFRvIII enhance killing of glioblastoma and patient-derived glioblastoma stem cells. Sci Rep 5:11483

Hegi ME, Diserens AC, Godard S, Dietrich PY, Regli L, Ostermann S, Otten P, Van Melle G, de Tribolet N, Stupp R (2004) Clinical trial substantiates the predictive value of O-6-methylguanine-DNA methyltransferase promoter methylation in glioblastoma patients treated with temozolomide. Clin Cancer Res 10(6):1871–1874

Heinrich T, Rengstl B, Muik A, Petkova M, Schmid F, Wistinghausen R, Warner K, Crispatzu G, Hansmann ML, Herling M, von Laer D, Newrzela S (2013) Mature T-cell lymphomagenesis induced by retroviral insertional activation of Janus kinase 1. Mol Ther 21(6):1160–1168

Hoffmann D, Göhring G, Heuser M, Ganser A, Schambach A, Morgan MA (2016) Letter to the Editor: production of mature healthy hematopoietic cells from induced pluripotent stem cells derived from an AML diagnostic sample containing the t(8;21) translocation. Stem Cells 34 (3):797–799

Hoseini SS, Hapke M, Herbst J, Wedekind D, Baumann R, Heinz N, Schiedlmeier B, Vignali DA, van den Brink MR, Schambach A, Blazar BR, Sauer MG (2015) Inducible T-cell receptor expression in precursor T cells for leukemia control. Leukemia 29(7):1530–1542

Hübner J, Hoseini SS, Suerth JD, Hoffmann D, Maluski M, Herbst J, Maul H, Ghosh A, Eiz-Vesper B, Yuan Q, Ott M, Heuser M, Schambach A, Sauer MG (2016) Generation of genetically engineered precursor T cells from human umbilical cord blood using an optimized alpharetroviral vector platform. Mol Ther 24(7):1216–1226

Jinek M, Chylinski K, Fonfara I, Hauer M, Doudna JA, Charpentier E (2012) A programmable dual-RNA–guided DNA endonuclease in adaptive bacterial immunity. Science 337:816–821

John LB, Devaud C, Duong CP, Yong CS, Beavis PA, Haynes NM, Chow MT, Smyth MJ, Kershaw MH, Darcy PK (2013) Anti-PD-1 antibody therapy potently enhances the eradication of established tumors by gene-modified T cells. Clin Cancer Res 19(20):5636–5646

Kalos M, Levine BL, Porter DL, Katz S, Grupp SA, Bagg A, June CH (2011) T cells with chimeric antigen receptors have potent antitumor effects and can establish memory in patients with advanced leukemia. Sci Transl Med 3(95):95ra73

Karlsson H, Svensson E, Gigg C, Jarvius M, Olsson-Strömberg U, Savoldo B, Dotti G, Loskog A (2015) Evaluation of intracellular signaling downstream chimeric antigen receptors. PLoS ONE 10(12):e0144787

Kaufmann KB, Brendel C, Suerth JD, Mueller-Kuller U, Chen-Wichmann L, Schwäble J, Pahujani S, Kunkel H, Schambach A, Baum C, Grez M (2013) Alpharetroviral vector-mediated gene therapy for X-CGD: functional correction and lack of aberrant splicing. Mol Ther 21 (3):648–661

Klco JM, Spencer DH, Miller CA, Griffith M, Lamprecht TL, O'Laughlin M, Fronick C, Magrini V, Demeter RT, Fulton RS, Eades WC, Link DC, Graubert TA, Walter MJ, Mardis ER, Dipersio JF, Wilson RK, Ley TJ (2014) Functional heterogeneity of genetically defined subclones in acute myeloid leukemia. Cancer Cell 25(3):379–392

Koike-Yusa H, Li Y, Tan EP, Velasco-Herrera Mdel C, Yusa K (2014) Genome-wide recessive genetic screening in mammalian cells with a lentiviral CRISPR-guide RNA library. Nat Biotechnol 32(3):267–273

Komor AC, Kim YB, Packer MS, Zuris JA, Liu DR (2016) Programmable editing of a target base in genomic DNA without double-stranded DNA cleavage. Nature 533(7603):420–424

Labenski V, Suerth JD, Barczak E, Heckl D, Levy C, Bernadin O, Charpentier E, Williams DA, Fehse B, Verhoeyen E, Schambach A (2016) Alpharetroviral self-inactivating vectors produced by a superinfection-resistant stable packaging cell line allow genetic modification of primary human T lymphocytes. Biomaterials 97:97–109

Laliberté J, Marquez VE, Momparler RL (1992) Potent inhibitors for the deamination of cytosine arabinoside and 5-aza-2′-deoxycytidine by human cytidine deaminase. Cancer Chemother Pharmacol 30(1):7–11

Mahfouz RZ, Jankowska A, Ebrahem Q, Gu X, Visconte V, Tabarroki A, Terse P, Covey J, Chan K, Ling Y, Engelke KJ, Sekeres MA, Tiu R, Maciejewski J, Radivoyevitch T, Saunthararajah Y (2013) Increased CDA expression/activity in males contributes to decreased cytidine analog half-life and likely contributes to worse outcomes with 5-azacytidine or decitabine therapy. Clin Cancer Res 19(4):938–948

Maier P, Fleckenstein K, Li L, Laufs S, Zeller WJ, Baum C, Fruehauf S, Herskind C, Wenz F (2006) Overexpression of MDR1 using a retroviral vector differentially regulates genes involved in detoxification and apoptosis and confers radioprotection. Radiat Res 166(3):463–473

Maier P, Herskind C, Fleckenstein K, Spier I, Laufs S, Zeller WJ, Fruehauf S, Wenz F (2008) MDR1 gene transfer using a lentiviral SIN vector confers radioprotection to human $CD34^+$ hematopoietic progenitor cells. Radiat Res 169(3):301–310

Maude SL, Frey N, Shaw PA, Aplenc R, Barrett DM, Bunin NJ, Chew A, Gonzalez VE, Zheng Z, Lacey SF, Mahnke YD, Melenhorst JJ, Rheingold SR, Shen A, Teachey DT, Levine BL, June CH, Porter DL, Grupp SA (2014) Chimeric antigen receptor T cells for sustained remissions in leukemia. N Engl J Med 371(16):1507–1517

Maze R, Kurpad C, Pegg AE, Erickson LC, Williams DA (1999) Retroviral-mediated expression of the P140A, but not P140A/G156A, mutant form of O6-methylguanine DNA methyltransferase protects hematopoietic cells against O6-benzylguanine sensitization to chloroethylnitrosourea treatment. J Pharmacol Exp Ther 290(3):1467–1474

Micucci F, Zingoni A, Piccoli M, Frati L, Santoni A, Galandrini R (2006) High-efficient lentiviral vector-mediated gene transfer into primary human NK cells. Exp Hematol 34:1344–1352

Mock U, Riecken K, Berdien B, Qasim W, Chan E, Cathomen T, Fehse B (2014) Novel lentiviral vectors with mutated reverse transcriptase for mRNA delivery of TALE nucleases. Sci Rep 4:6409

Moiani A, Suerth JD, Gandolfi F, Rizzi E, Severgnini M, De Bellis G, Schambach A, Mavilio F (2014) Genome-wide analysis of alpharetroviral integration in human hematopoietic stem/progenitor cells. Genes (Basel) 5(2):415–429

Moritz T, Mackay W, Glassner BJ, Williams DA, Samson L (1995) Retrovirus-mediated expression of a DNA repair protein in bone marrow protects hematopoietic cells from nitrosourea-induced toxicity in vitro and in vivo. Cancer Res 55(12):2608–2614

Naldini L (2015) Gene therapy returns to centre stage. Nature 526(7573):351–360

Namuduri M, Brentjens RJ (2016) Medical management of side effects related to CAR T cell therapy in hematologic malignancies. Expert Rev Hematol 19:1–3 (Epub ahead of print)

Newrzela S, Cornils K, Heinrich T, Schläger J, Yi JH, Lysenko O, Kimpel J, Fehse B, von Laer D (2011) Retroviral insertional mutagenesis can contribute to immortalization of mature T lymphocytes. Mol Med 17(11–12):1223–1232

Newrzela S, Al-Ghaili N, Heinrich T, Petkova M, Hartmann S, Rengstl B, Kumar A, Jäck HM, Gerdes S, Roeder I, Hansmann ML, von Laer D (2012) T-cell receptor diversity prevents T-cell lymphoma development. Leukemia 26(12):2499–2507

Ott MG, Schmidt M, Schwarzwaelder K, Stein S, Siler U, Koehl U, Glimm H, Kühlcke K, Schilz A, Kunkel H, Naundorf S, Brinkmann A, Deichmann A, Fischer M, Ball C, Pilz I, Dunbar C, Du Y, Jenkins NA, Copeland NG, Lüthi U, Hassan M, Thrasher AJ, Hoelzer D, von Kalle C, Seger R, Grez M (2006) Correction of X-linked chronic granulomatous disease by gene therapy, augmented by insertional activation of MDS1-EVI1, PRDM16 or SETBP1. Nat Med 12(4):401–409

Pardoll DM (2012) The blockade of immune checkpoints in cancer immunotherapy. Nat Rev Cancer 12(4):252–264

Porter DL, Hwang WT, Frey NV, Lacey SF, Shaw PA, Loren AW, Bagg A, Marcucci KT, Shen A, Gonzalez V, Ambrose D, Grupp SA, Chew A, Zheng Z, Milone MC, Levine BL, Melenhorst JJ, June CH (2015) Chimeric antigen receptor T cells persist and induce sustained remissions in relapsed refractory chronic lymphocytic leukemia. Sci Transl Med 7 (303):303ra139

Rapoport AP, Stadtmauer EA, Binder-Scholl GK, Goloubeva O, Vogl DT, Lacey SF, Badros AZ, Garfall A, Weiss B, Finklestein J, Kulikovskaya I, Sinha SK, Kronsberg S, Gupta M, Bond S, Melchiori L, Brewer JE, Bennett AD, Gerry AB, Pumphrey NJ, Williams D, Tayton-Martin HK, Ribeiro L, Holdich T, Yanovich S, Hardy N, Yared J, Kerr N, Philip S, Westphal S, Siegel DL, Levine BL, Jakobsen BK, Kalos M, June CH (2015) NY-ESO-1-specific TCR-engineered T cells mediate sustained antigen-specific antitumor effects in myeloma. Nat Med 21(8):914–921

Robbins PF, Kassim SH, Tran TL, Crystal JS, Morgan RA, Feldman SA, Yang JC, Dudley ME, Wunderlich JR, Sherry RM, Kammula US, Hughes MS, Restifo NP, Raffeld M, Lee CC, Li YF, El-Gamil M, Rosenberg SA (2015) A pilot trial using lymphocytes genetically engineered with an NY-ESO-1-reactive T-cell receptor: long-term follow-up and correlates with response. Clin Cancer Res 21(5):1019–10127

Ruan H, Qiu S, Beard BC, Black ME (2016) Creation of zebularine-resistant human cytidine deaminase mutants to enhance the chemoprotection of hematopoietic stem cells. Protein Eng Des Sel May 8. pii: gzw012 (Epub ahead of print)

Salci KR, Lee JH, Laronde S, Dingwall S, Kushwah R, Fiebig-Comyn A, Leber B, Foley R, Dal Cin A, Bhatia M (2015) Cellular reprogramming allows generation of autologous hematopoietic progenitors from AML patients that are devoid of patient-specific genomic aberrations. Stem Cells 33(6):1839–1849

Sánchez-Rivera FJ, Papagiannakopoulos T, Romero R, Tammela T, Bauer MR, Bhutkar A, Joshi NS, Subbaraj L, Bronson RT, Xue W, Jacks T (2014) Rapid modelling of cooperating genetic events in cancer through somatic genome editing. Nature 516(7531):428–431

Sancho-Martinez I, Nivet E, Xia Y, Hishida T, Aguirre A, Ocampo A, Ma L, Morey R, Krause MN, Zembrzycki A, Ansorge O, Vazquez-Ferrer E, Dubova I, Reddy P, Lam D, Hishida Y, Wu MZ, Esteban CR, O'Leary D, Wahl GM, Verma IM, Laurent LC, Izpisua Belmonte JC (2016) Establishment of human iPSC-based models for the study and targeting of glioma initiating cells. Nat Commun 7:10743. doi:10.1038/ncomms10743

Sandri S, Bobisse S, Moxley K, Lamolinara A, De Sanctis F, Boschi F, Sbarbati A, Fracasso G, Ferrarini G, Hendriks RW, Cavallini C, Scupoli MT, Sartoris S, Iezzi M, Nishimura MI, Bronte V, Ugel S (2016) Feasibility of telomerase-specific adoptive T-cell therapy for B-cell chronic lymphocytic leukemia and solid malignancies. Cancer Res 76(9):2540–2551

Schambach A, Schiedlmeier B, Kühlcke K, Verstegen M, Margison GP, Li Z, Kamino K, Bohne J, Alexandrov A, Hermann FG, von Laer D, Baum C (2006) Towards hematopoietic stem cell-mediated protection against infection with human immunodeficiency virus. Gene Ther 13 (13):1037–1047

Schröder JK, Kirch C, Seeber S, Schütte J (1998) Structural and functional analysis of the cytidine deaminase gene in patients with acute myeloid leukaemia. Br J Haematol 103(4):1096–1103

Scott AM, Wolchok JD, Old LJ (2012) Antibody therapy of cancer. Nat Rev Cancer 12(4):278–287

Shalem O, Sanjana NE, Hartenian E, Shi X, Scott DA, Mikkelsen TS, Heckl D, Ebert BL, Root DE, Doench JG, Zhang F (2014) Genome-scale CRISPR-Cas9 knockout screening in human cells. Science 343(6166):84–87

Shen DW, Fojo A, Chin JE, Roninson IB, Richert N, Pastan I, Gottesman MM (1986) Human multidrug-resistant cell lines: increased mdr1 expression can precede gene amplification. Science 232(4750):643–645

Singh N, Frey NV, Grupp SA, Maude SL (2016) CAR T cell therapy in acute lymphoblastic leukemia and potential for chronic lymphocytic leukemia. Curr Treat Options Oncol 17(6):28

Spary LK, Al-Taei S, Salimu J, Cook AD, Ager A, Watson HA, Clayton A, Staffurth J, Mason MD, Tabi Z (2014) Enhancement of T cell responses as a result of synergy between lower doses of radiation and T cell stimulation. J Immunol 192(7):3101–3110

Straathof KC, Pule MA, Yotnda P, Dotti G, Vanin EF, Brenner MK, Heslop HE, Spencer DM, Rooney CM (2005) An inducible caspase 9 safety switch for T-cell therapy. Blood 105:4247–4254

Suerth JD, Maetzig T, Brugman MH, Heinz N, Appelt JU, Kaufmann KB, Schmidt M, Grez M, Modlich U, Baum C, Schambach A (2012) Alpharetroviral self-inactivating vectors: long-term transgene expression in murine hematopoietic cells and low genotoxicity. Mol Ther 20 (5):1022–1032

Suerth JD, Morgan MA, Kloess S, Heckl D, Neudörfl C, Falk CS, Koehl U, Schambach A (2016) Efficient generation of gene-modified human natural killer cells via alpharetroviral vectors. J Mol Med (Berl) 94(1):83–93

Takahashi K, Yamanaka S (2006) Induction of pluripotent stem cells from mouse embryonic and adult fibroblast cultures by defined factors. Cell 126:663–676

Tano K, Shiota S, Collier J, Foote RS, Mitra S (1990) Isolation and structural characterization of a cDNA clone encoding the human DNA repair protein for O6-alkylguanine. Proc Natl Acad Sci USA 87(2):686–690

Töpfer K, Cartellieri M, Michen S, Wiedemuth R, Müller N, Lindemann D, Bachmann M, Füssel M, Schackert G, Temme A (2015) DAP12-based activating chimeric antigen receptor for NK cell tumor immunotherapy. J Immunol 194(7):3201–3212

Uchiyama T, Adriani M, Jagadeesh GJ, Paine A, Candotti F (2012) Foamy virus vector-mediated gene correction of a mouse model of Wiskott-Aldrich syndrome. Mol Ther 20(6):1270–1279

van der Merwe PA, Davis SJ (2003) Molecular interactions mediating T cell antigen recognition. Annu Rev Immunol 21:659–684

van Rhee F, Szmania SM, Zhan F, Gupta SK, Pomtree M, Lin P, Batchu RB, Moreno A, Spagnoli G, Shaughnessy J, Tricot G (2005) NY-ESO-1 is highly expressed in poor-prognosis multiple myeloma and induces spontaneous humoral and cellular immune responses. Blood 105(10):3939–3944

Vogelstein B, Papadopoulos N, Velculescu VE, Zhou S, Diaz LA Jr, Kinzler KW (2013) Cancer genome landscapes. Science 339(6127):1546–1558

Vogler I, Newrzela S, Hartmann S, Schneider N, von Laer D, Koehl U, Grez M (2010) An improved bicistronic CD20/tCD34 vector for efficient purification and *in vivo* depletion of gene-modified T cells for adoptive immunotherapy. Mol Ther 18:1330–1338

Wang X, Chang WC, Wong CW, Colcher D, Sherman M, Ostberg JR, Forman SJ, Riddell SR, Jensen MC (2011) A transgene-encoded cell surface polypeptide for selection, in vivo tracking, and ablation of engineered cells. Blood 118:1255–1263

Wang J, Li T, Zhou M, Hu Z, Zhou X, Zhou S, Wang N, Huang L, Zhao L, Cao Y, Xiao M, Ma D, Zhou P, Shang Z, Zhou J (2015) TALENs-mediated gene disruption of FLT3 in leukemia cells: using genome-editing approach for exploring the molecular basis of gene abnormality. Sci Rep 5:18454

Zhang C, Burger MC, Jennewein L, Genßler S, Schönfeld K, Zeiner P, Hattingen E, Harter PN, Mittelbronn M, Tonn T, Steinbach JP, Wels WS (2016) ErbB2/HER2-specific NK cells for targeted therapy of glioblastoma. J Natl Cancer Inst 108(5). pii: djv375. doi:10.1093/jnci/djv375

Zhu Y, Tan Y, Ou R, Zhong Q, Zheng L, Du Y, Zhang Q, Huang J (2016) Anti-CD19 chimeric antigen receptor-modified T cells for B-cell malignancies: a systematic review of efficacy and safety in clinical trials. Eur J Haematol 96(4):389–396

Minicircle-Based Engineering of Chimeric Antigen Receptor (CAR) T Cells

Michael Hudecek, Tea Gogishvili, Razieh Monjezi, Julia Wegner, Ram Shankar, Christa Kruesemann, Csaba Miskey, Zoltán Ivics, Marco Schmeer and Martin Schleef

Abstract

Plasmid DNA is being used as a pharmaceutical agent in vaccination, as well as a basic substance and starting material in gene and cell therapy, and viral vector production. Since the uncontrolled expression of backbone sequences present in such plasmids and the dissemination of antibiotic resistance genes may have profound detrimental effects, an important goal in vector development was to produce supercoiled DNA lacking bacterial backbone sequences: *Minicircle* (MC) DNA. The *Sleeping Beauty* (SB) transposon system is a non-viral gene delivery platform enabling a close-to-random profile of genomic integration. In combination, the MC platform greatly enhances SB transposition and transgene integration resulting in higher numbers of stably modified target cells. We have recently developed a strategy for MC-based SB transposition of chimeric antigen receptor (CAR) transgenes that enable improved transposition rates compared to conventional plasmids and rapid manufacturing of therapeutic CAR T cell doses (Monjezi et al. 2016). This advance enables manufacturing CAR T cells in a virus-free process that relies on SB-mediated transposition from MC DNA to accomplish gene-transfer. Advantages of this approach include a strong safety profile due to the nature of the MC itself and the genomic insertion pattern of MC-derived CAR transposons. In addition, stable transposition and high-level CAR transgene expression, as well as easy and reproducible handling, make MCs a preferred vector source for gene-transfer in advanced cellular and gene

M. Hudecek · T. Gogishvili · R. Monjezi · J. Wegner
Medizinische Klinik und Poliklinik II, Universitätsklinikum Würzburg, Würzburg, Germany

R. Shankar · C. Kruesemann · M. Schmeer · M. Schleef (✉)
PlasmidFactory, Bielefeld, Germany
e-mail: martin.schleef@plasmidfactory.com

C. Miskey · Z. Ivics
Division of Medical Biotechnology, Paul-Ehrlich-Institute, Langen, Germany

W. Walther (ed.), *Current Strategies in Cancer Gene Therapy*,
Recent Results in Cancer Research 209, DOI 10.1007/978-3-319-42934-2_3

therapy. In this chapter, we will review our experience in MC-based CAR T cell engineering and discuss our recent advances in MC manufacturing to accelerate both pre-clinical and clinical implementation.

Keywords
Sleeping Beauty · Minicircle · Transposition · Chimeric antigen receptor T cell · Immunotherapy

1 Introduction

1.1 MC DNA as Minimalistic Expression Cassette

MCs are derived from parental plasmid (PP) with antibiotic resistance marker, the gene of interest (GOI) and *ori*, as well as two special signal sequences right and left of the GOI. Through an intramolecular recombination process, the GOI (plus one of the recombination and purification sequence elements, SCAR) is cut out of that parental plasmid, circularized, and finally results in only the GOI and the signal sequence in a supercoiled (ccc) circular molecule.

Several recombinases have earlier been used so far to achieve this intramolecular recombination process: the integrase of bacteriophage lambda, the Cre recombinase from bacteriophage P1, the FLP recombinase of the yeast plasmid 2-μm circle, and the integrase of Streptomyces bacteriophage PhiC31 or the ParA resolvase from the multimer resolution system of the broad host range plasmid RK2 or RP4 (Bigger et al. 2001; Chen et al. 2003; Darquet et al. 1997; Jechlinger et al. 2004; Nehlsen et al. 2006) to separate the parental plasmid (PP) into a miniplasmid (MP) and a MC [a comprehensive overview was given by Schleef (2013)].

In earlier work, the ParA resolvase, a serine recombinase that mediates an intramolecular recombination between corresponding directly repeated resolution sites (Eberl et al. 1994; Smith and Thorpe 2002; Thomson and Ow 2006) in exclusively one direction to completion, is working successfully. Hence, a supercoiled monomeric MC is obtained (Jechlinger et al. 2004).

For successful MC production, an efficient silencing of recombinase expression before induction is important to avoid early recombination events leading to the displacement of the parental plasmid by the miniplasmid, that still contains the bacterial *ori*, hence replicating in bacteria. The P BAD/araC arabinose expression system (Bigger et al. 2001; Chen et al. 2003; Jechlinger et al. 2004) has been shown to be able to inhibit background expression of the recombinases in the noninduced state.

After successful recombination, the MC has to be isolated from a mixture of three types of circular DNA molecules: MCs, miniplasmids, and maybe residual amounts of parental plasmids. This is done by a set of chromatography steps, including a tailor-made affinity chromatography step. The approach to selectively bind a sequence motif (identification sequence part of SCAR) with the purpose of separating this from a mixture of different DNAs (Gossen et al. 1993) led to the approach that we initially published in 2008 (Mayrhofer et al. 2008; Schleef and Schmeer 2011; Schleef et al. 2015).

Besides fulfilling requirements concerning product safety, MCs show a significantly higher efficiency with respect to gene expression levels and duration in vitro and in vivo, making them useful tools for future therapeutic applications (Kobelt et al. 2013; Chabot et al. 2013), and were recently presented the first time allowing the production of AAV particles, free of antibiotic resistance, and other prokaryotic sequence motifs.

1.2 Non-viral Gene-Transfer Through *Sleeping Beauty* Transposition

SB transposons enable close-to-random integration into the genome of mammalian (Izsvak et al. 2010; Ivics and Izsvak 2011; Aronovich et al. 2011; Swierczek et al. 2012). SB was derived from an ancient, inactive transposon from several fish genomes. After various modifications, a hyperactive transposase (SB100) could be developed that yields enhanced stable gene-transfer in several human cell types including T cells (Ivics et al. 1997; Mates et al. 2009). The potential to use SB-mediated transposition to integrate CAR and T cell receptor transgenes in human T cells has been intensively investigated (Izsvak et al. 2010; Swierczek et al. 2012; Peng et al. 2009; Field et al. 2013; Huang et al. 2008; Jin et al. 2011; Singh et al. 2008, 2013, 2014). Nevertheless, transfection of conventional plasmid DNA to provide transposon and transposase typically resulted in low gene-transfer rates and extensive T cell toxicity, and hence, long ex vivo culture times were required to generate therapeutic doses of gene-modified T cells.

The SB gene-transfer strategy is based on mobile genetic elements, the transposons, containing a gene of interest flanked by inverted terminal repeats (IR/DR), and a transposase that binds to the IR/DR and mobilizes the transposon for integration into the target genome through a cut-and-paste mechanism. Those two elements are typically encoded on two separate vectors. Alternatively, the transposase can be encoded by an RNA molecule, while the transposable element (the gene of interest—GOI—to be integrated into the genome of the target cell) is still encoded on a DNA molecule. As initially presented by Izsvak et al. (2010), the structure of this transposon molecule is influencing the transposition efficacy. While the proximal sequences between the IR/DR are to be transposed, the other (distal) sequences between the IR/DRs (in other words the residual molecule "behind" the IR/DR) are remaining outside the genome of the modified cell and are expected to be subject of degradation.

1.3 Principles of CAR Design

Adoptive immunotherapy with gene-engineered tumor-reactive T cells expressing a transgenic T cell receptor (TCR) or synthetic CAR is emerging as a powerful and potentially curative treatment of malignant diseases. CARs are fusion proteins comprised of an extracellular antigen-binding domain, most commonly a single-chain variable fragment (scFv) of variable heavy (VH) and variable light (VL) chains of a monoclonal antibody, and an intracellular signaling module. To link the extracellular and intracellular portion, various spacer and transmembrane (TM) domains are used that anchor the receptor on the T cell surface. The signaling module of first-generation CARs contained only the CD3ζ chain (Signal 1), and second- and third-generation CARs include one or two (respectively) costimulatory domains, e.g., CD28, 4-1BB, OX40, or ICOS, to provide Signal 2 which is critical for optimal T cell stimulation and induction of an effective immune response (reviewed in: Turtle et al. 2012).

A key difference of CAR recognition, compared to the TCR, is the ability of CARs to bind to surface molecules on target cells. Thus, CAR recognition does not depend on the intracellular processing of antigens and presentation of immunogenic peptides on HLA (human leukocyte antigen) molecules. Another important aspect is that CARs as synthetic molecules can be equipped with targeting domains that bind not only to proteins but also to a broad range of potential tumor targets such as carbohydrates, gangliosides, proteoglycans, and also heavily glycosylated proteins, expanding the panel of antigens that can be targeted on tumor cells.

1.4 Gene-Transfer Strategies and Clinical Experience with CAR T Cells

There are two principle strategies for expressing the CAR transgene in T cells: (i) transiently, e.g., by transfection of CAR-encoding mRNA, which provides a window of activity in the range of several days and is self-limiting by the fading expression of receptor and dilution of the mRNA as the T cells start to proliferate (Beatty et al. 2014) and (ii) permanently by stable gene-transfer with viral or non-viral vectors. The majority of pre-clinical and clinical work with CAR T cells is performed using stable gene-transfer, and the overwhelming majority of investigators is using gamma-retroviral (RV) and lentiviral vectors (LV) for gene-transfer (reviewed in: Ramos et al. 2014). The use of non-viral gene-transfer by SB-mediated transposition for CAR T cell engineering has been explored but was limited by very low gene-transfer rates and significant toxicity to T cells after transfection of conventional plasmids to insert SB transposase and CAR transposon (Singh et al. 2008, 2013; Field et al. 2013). We have recently shown that both challenges can be addressed by the use of MCs to encode SB transposase and transposon (Monjezi et al. 2016). Table 1 provides a comparison of key features of LV- and SB-mediated gene-transfer.

Table 1 Summary of key features of viral vectors and SB MC vector used as gene-transfer vehicles

Gene delivery vector	Viral vectors	*Sleeping Beauty* MC vector
Host range	Broad	Broad
Gene-transfer efficiency	High	High
Transgene expression stability	Long-term	Long-term
Immunogenicity	Yes	NA
Genotoxicity/insertional mutagenesis	Yes	NA
Vector integration site profile	Bias to oncogenes/exons/highly expressed genes, 3 % to GSH	Close to random, 23 % to GSH
Transgenic capacity size	Low to high (<4 kbp to >30 kbp)	Not known upper limit
Storage and handling	Special caution required	No special caution required
Cost of production	High	NA

NA Data not available
GSH Genomic safe harbor

A critical issue in cancer immunotherapy is to identify target antigens that allow selective (or preferential) elimination of tumor cells while sparing normal tissues. The clinical development of CAR T cell therapy is most advanced in hematologic malignancies, i.e., B cell leukemia and lymphoma with CARs targeting the B cell marker CD19. An anticipated but acceptable side effect of CD19-CAR therapy is the depletion of normal B cells. Coexpression of "safety switches," e.g., a truncated epidermal growth factor receptor (EGFRt) depletion marker (Wang et al. 2011) or inducible caspase-9 (iCasp9) suicide genes (Di Stasi et al. 2011), can be used to delete CAR T cells after a therapeutic window to prevent, terminate, or mitigate undesired effects or toxicity of CAR T cells.

Most of currently reported pre-clinical and clinical studies with CAR T cells employ bulk CD3+ T cells that contain a random composition of naïve and memory CD8+ killer, CD4+ helper, and potentially even CD4+ regulatory T cell subsets. All of these T cell subsets are not only phenotypically, but also functionally distinct, and their frequency differs substantially between individuals. Thus, there is significant product to product heterogeneity in cell composition when CAR T cell is prepared from a bulk CD3+ T cell population (Brentjens et al. 2011). This heterogeneity complicates the analysis and interpretation of data obtained in pre-clinical experiments and in the clinical setting, as essentially every patient is receiving a cell product of different potency and with different attributes in pharmacokinetic and -dynamic. Therefore, we prefer to perform CAR gene-transfer into defined T cell subsets (in the easiest case, separately into CD8+ killer and CD4+ helper T cells), analyze their in vitro function separately in our pre-clinical models, and formulate CAR T cell products with defined CD8+ and CD4+ subset

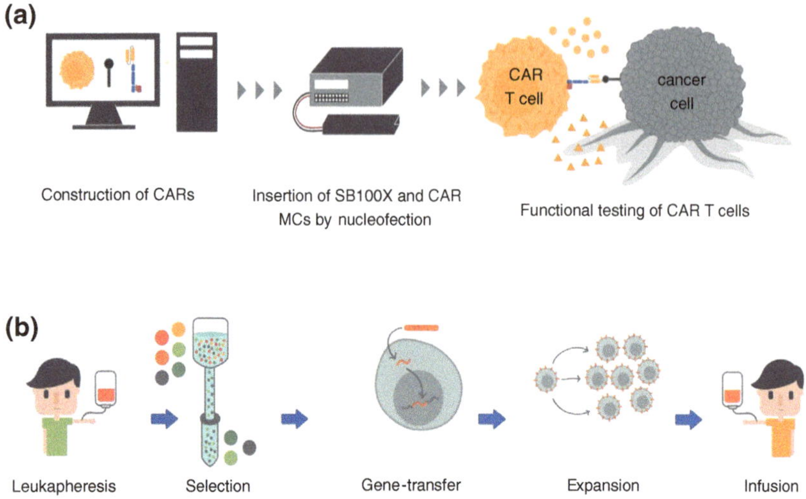

Fig. 1 **a** CARs are designed using specialized computer software. MCs encoding the genetic information for the CAR are introduced into T cells using a nucleofector. CAR T cell effector functions such as cytolytic activity, cytokine secretion, and proliferation are tested in pre-clinical models. **b** To prepare CAR T cells, white blood cells are harvested in a process called leukapheresis and appropriate T cell subsets (e.g., CD8+ killer and CD4+ helper T cells) are purified. Gene-transfer is performed using MC-encoded SB100X transposase and CAR transposon. CAR T cells are expanded prior to administration to patient

composition for in vivo studies and clinical applications Fig. 1a. We have recently shown that this strategy is advantageous to the use of bulk CD3+ T cells and have successfully translated this concept into the clinical setting (Sommermeyer et al. 2016; Turtle et al. 2016). The CAR T cell manufacturing process is summarized in Fig. 1b.

2 Methodologies of SB-Minicircle and CAR T Cell Manufacturing

2.1 Construction of Transposable MC Vectors

The existing and functionally evaluated plasmid encoding SB100, also known as SB100X (Ivics et al. 1997), was used to purify a restriction fragment to transfer into the parental plasmid (PP) in a way that after recombination of MC induction, the SB100 expression cassette is located on the resulting MC (Fig. 2a). This was carried out by inserting a BglII restriction fragment of the plasmid pcDNA3.1-CMV-SB100, carrying the SB100 expression cassette, into the BglII restriction site of the parental plasmid PP11 published earlier (Schleef et al. 2015). The resulting pP11.SB100 contains the SB100 expression cassette and a sequence tag for the

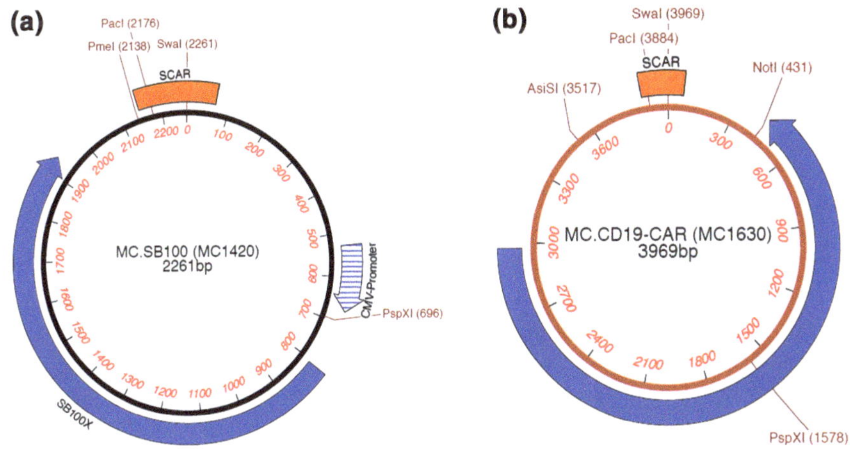

Fig. 2 *Minicircle* DNAs for SB100 (**a**) and for CD19-CAR (**b**), consisting only of the GOI plus one of the recombination and purification sequence elements (SCAR) as a supercoiled (ccc) circular molecule

subsequent purification of MC.SB100, flanked by the recombination sequences. Importantly, no backbone sequences (e.g., bacterial origin of replication and selection marker) are contained within this area. Such sequences are positioned outside the framed area and will finally end up on the miniplasmid as by-product and are removed during affinity chromatography. The resulting MC and miniplasmid both contain the recombination sequence. The remaining nucleotides of recombination and tag sequences on the MC are called "SCAR" (sequence for chromatography, affinity, and recombination) since they constitute the only small portion on the MC that is neither the part of the expression cassette nor the GOI.

A CD19-CAR-encoding MC was derived from a parental pT2HB_CD19-CAR plasmid and obtained by inserting the restriction fragment with the CD19-CAR gene into the PP in a way that also in this case, the resulting MC carries the CD19-CAR gene (Fig. 2b). This was carried out by transferring the Eco53kI and SalI restriction fragment of pT2HB_CD19-CAR into the parental plasmid PP11 (see above) resulting in a parental plasmid pP11.CD19-CAR. This PP was also subject to recombination to obtain MC and miniplasmid as described in detail above.

2.2 Manufacturing of MC DNA

The production of the two MC DNAs for SB100 and for CD19-CAR used in this publication (performed as a service of PlasmidFactory, Bielefeld, Germany) was carried out in 2 major production steps: the microbial cultivation in a bioreactor and the purification by specific chromatographic steps. The cultivations of *E. coli* cells carrying the respective parental plasmids were carried out at 37 °C in a MBR bioreactor (MBR BIO REACTOR, Switzerland) with 5 L, pH adjusted to 7.0 with

2 M sodium hydroxide solution and 2 M phosphoric acid. The airflow rate was fixed at 5 L/min. The oxygen concentration of 60 % was controlled by varying the stirrer speed. LB medium was used without addition of any antibiotics and free of any substance deriving from any animal source. The bioreactor was inoculated with 50 mL of an *E. coli* K12 culture transformed with the parental plasmid PP and grown in LB medium (as pre-culture) for approximately 15 h. Recombinase expression was induced at an OD_{600} » 4 by adding L-arabinose. After an additional 1 h of growth, cells were harvested by centrifugation, frozen, and purified.

The recombination product (MC and miniplasmid) was further purified after the primary recovery as presented earlier (Mayrhofer et al. 2008) with a modified non-commercial proprietary chromatography matrix obtained from PlasmidFactory (Bielefeld, Germany). The specific binding of MC DNA was optimized with different ionic strength and pH values and resulted in a highly purified product as shown below.

2.3 Engineering of CAR T Cells

CD8+ killer and CD4+ helper T cells were isolated from Peripheral blood mononuclear cells (PBMC) were isolated from heparinized peripheral blood by centrifugation over Ficoll-Paque. Distinct T cell subsets were obtained by negative selection using magnetic microbeads (Miltenyi, Bergisch-Gladbach, Germany) or reversible Streptamers® that mark the target cell population but can subsequently be released with biotin to yield quasi-untouched T cells (IBA, Göttingen, Germany). The purity and yield of the T cell population was determined by flow cytometry using conjugated mAbs specific for CD3, CD4, and CD8. 7-AAD (BD Biosciences, San Jose, CA) was used to discriminate dead from live cells.

Although SB transposition can be directly performed in freshly isolated T cells, we observed that gene-transfer rates are substantially higher, and the subsequent expansion of T cells much more productive, if prior T cell activation is performed. T cells can be activated through anti-CD3/CD28 stimulation using Dynabeads (ThermoFisher, Waltham, MA) for 2 days prior to SB transposition or by culture on anti-CD3/CD28 mAb-coated plates. T cells were propagated in RPMI-1640 medium supplemented with 10 % human serum, glutamine, 100 U/mL penicillin–streptomycin, and 50 U/mL recombinant human IL-2.

Transfection of SB100 and CAR-encoding MC can be accomplished by electroporation. We performed nucleofection using a 4D nucleofector (Lonza, Cologne, Germany): 1–2 × 10e6 of activated T cells were nucleofected with 1 μg of each transposon and transposase conventional plasmids or equimolar amount of their corresponding MC DNA vectors in 20 μl of P3 primary cell line buffer based on manufacturer's protocol (Lonza). T cell viability was monitored by trypan blue staining. The EGFRt transduction marker that is encoded *in cis* with the CAR in the SB transposon was utilized to detect and enrich CAR+ (i.e., EGFRt+) T cells prior to expansion with irradiated CD19+ feeder cells and functional testing (Hudecek et al. 2013, 2015). Functional analyses aim at documenting the specificity of

CAR T cells for the targeted tumor antigen and the ability to eliminate tumor cells. Functional testing is preceded and accompanied by careful phenotypic analysis of the CAR T cell product by flow cytometry including CD3, CD4, and CD8, expression of the CAR transgene (using the EGFRt marker).

2.4 Functional Testing of CAR T Cells

In vitro characterization of CAR T cells typically focuses on the 3 cardinal effector functions—cytolytic activity, cytokine production, and proliferation. The specific cytolytic effect against relevant target cells, i.e., CD19+ lymphoma cell lines, and CD19− control targets, was analyzed in a 4-h bioluminescence-based cytotoxicity assay (Brown et al. 2005). The assay was set up in triplicate wells of a 96-well plate at effector:target cell ratios ranging from 20:1 to 1:1, using 5000 target cells per well. The specific lysis of CD19+ target cells was calculated using the standard formula (Brown et al. 2005). The production of cytokines such as IFNg and IL-2 was analyzed in supernatants that were removed from cocultures of 50,000 CAR-transduced and control untransduced T cells with target cells (effector:target cell ratio: 4:1 to 2:1) after 20 h of incubation. Cytokines were quantified by ELISA or multiplex cytokine analysis. Antigen-dependent induction of CAR T cell proliferation was evaluated by CFSE dye dilution after 72 h of coculture of effector and target cells, and finally the viability of CAR T cells was analyzed by 7-AAD staining.

For pre-clinical in vivo studies, xenograft models in immunodeficient NSG mice (NOD-Scid-gc$^{-/-}$) are well established and have been demonstrated to provide clinically relevant data on antitumor efficacy, as well as on CAR T cell engraftment and persistence. We performed analyses in NSG mice that were engrafted with 0.5–1 × 10e6 firefly-luciferase transduced Raji lymphoma cells. Raji was inoculated by tail vein injection and mice treated with CAR-modified or unmodified T cells on day 7, when systemic lymphoma had developed. The antitumor response was analyzed by serial bioluminescence imaging after administration of D-luciferin substrate (IVIS Lumina, Perkin-Elmer, Waltham, MA) (Hudecek et al. 2013, 2015; Monjezi et al. 2016).

3 Antitumor Function of Minicircle Engineered CAR T Cells

3.1 Characterization of MC DNA

The plasmid and MC DNA used to perform the experiments presented here were characterized by a comprehensive QC. The content of LPS-endotoxin was determined at <20 E.U./mg by the use of a Kinetic-QCL kit (Lonza), the DNA concentration was adjusted to 1 mg/mL, and the DNA was dissolved in water for injection (WFI). CGE and agarose gel date could demonstrate that the products each were pure and predominantly a homogenous supercoiled MC DNA (Fig. 3).

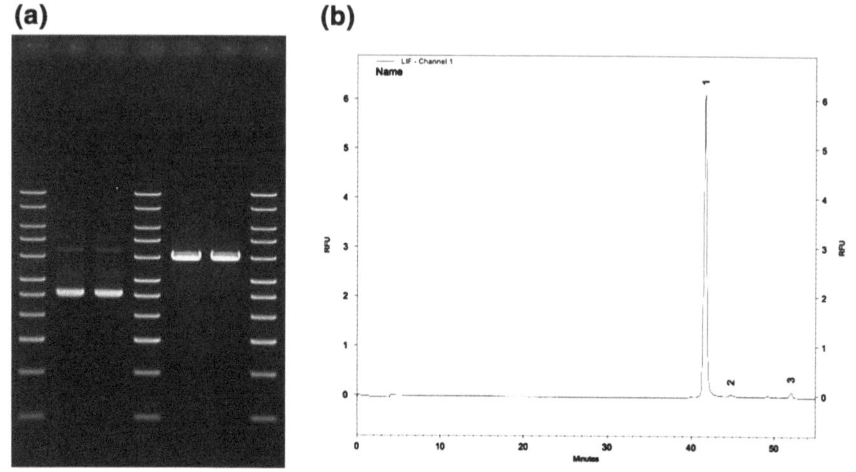

Fig. 3 **a** 0.8 % agarose gel electrophoresis stained with ethidium bromide after gel run (1 V/cm) of the circular, supercoiled, monomeric MC.CD19-CAR (lanes 2 and 3) and the linearization product (lanes 5 and 6; PacI digest resulting in a 3969 bp fragment). 1 kbp ladder in lanes 1, 4, and 7 (PlasmidFactory, item no. MSM-865-50). **b** Capillary gel electrophoresis of the circular, supercoiled (ccc), monomeric MC MC.CD19-CAR (peak 1; 97.3 %). Peak 2 (1.2 %) and peak 3 (1.5 %) are traces of relaxed circular (rc) and open circular (oc) molecules

3.2 Gene-Transfer Rate and Integration Profile

We have recently shown that high-level, stable gene-transfer can be accomplished by cotransfection of MC-encoded SB100 and CD19-CAR in both CD8+ and CD4+ T cells (Monjezi et al. 2016). Stable gene-transfer rates of >50 % can routinely be accomplished with MCs and are typically slightly higher in CD4+ compared to CD8+ T cells. Importantly, the gene-transfer rate after cotransfection of MCs is significantly higher compared to corresponding conventional plasmids, and the process less toxic, most likely due to the lower amount of DNA that is introduced into T cells. Whether or not transient gene expression can be obtained by transfection of transgene-encoding MC alone (i.e., without SB100X) depends on the amount of MC that is being transfected and varies considerably between transgenes.

Genome-wide insertion site analysis is an approach to assess genotoxicity associated with genetic modification. We analyzed insertion sites of CD19-CAR transposons that had been mobilized from MCs to determine whether there was a preference for integration into distinct sites of the genome. For CD19-CAR transposons, mobilized from MCs as described in this chapter, we detected a close-to-random integration profile, without preference for highly expressed or cancer-related genes (Monjezi et al. 2016). Thus, the previously described, favorable integration pattern of SB was well maintained, even though the gene-transfer rate with MCs was substantially higher than in previous studies with conventional plasmid DNA. Criteria have been defined that identify "genomic safe harbor" (GSH) where integration is neither expected to cause genotoxicity, nor malignant transformation (Sadelain et al. 2011). A comprehensive GSH analysis disclosed a significantly higher percentage of GSH integrations had occurred with SB transposons after mobilization from MCs compared to LV integrants. These attributes make SB transposition from MCs the most effective and safest stable gene-transfer strategy known to date.

3.3 Functional Characterization of CAR T Cells

CAR T cells that were engineered with MC-based SB transposition displayed specific and very potent effector functions in vitro and in pre-clinical models in vivo (Monjezi et al. 2016). Importantly, CAR expression and CAR T cell antitumor function were stable over several weeks and multiple rounds of expansion, confirming that mobilization of the CAR transposon from the MC had resulted in stable integration and high-level transgene expression without gene silencing. We have also demonstrated in vitro and in vivo that the antitumor function of CAR T cells that we engineered by SB transposition from MCs was equally potent as with CAR T cells that were generated from the same donors by lentiviral gene-transfer (Monjezi et al. 2016). This is encouraging, and efforts to obtain clinical validation for the potency and safety of adoptive therapy with MC-engineered CAR T cells are ongoing.

The function of CAR T cells is influenced by the copy number of the CAR gene in their genome. The current paradigm is that higher gene copy number leads to higher expression of CAR protein and potentially better function, although an upper threshold may be reached where the expression of the CAR on the T cell surface and availability of adaptor proteins that propagate CAR signaling are saturated, or where the signal of the CAR is getting too strong and induces activation-induced cell death (AICD). We have shown that the number of CD19-CAR transposons in T cells that were transfected with MC-encoded SB100 transposase and CAR transposon correlates with the expression of CAR and EGFRt protein and is well balanced between CD8+ and CD4+ T cells, and in a similar range as the number of LV integrants after viral gene-transfer (Monjezi et al. 2016). Further, a comprehensive integration site analysis of CAR transposons demonstrated that a significantly higher proportion of integrations had occurred in GSH that is not expected to cause genotoxicity or malignant transformation (Monjezi et al. 2016). Intriguingly, the use of MC DNA for CAR gene-transfer provides the opportunity to use titrated amounts of MC during gene-transfer until a gene copy number has been reached that is optimal with regard to gene-transfer rate and CAR T cell function and satisfactory for regulators with regard to transposon copy number and number of GSH integrations.

4 Future Perspectives

4.1 GMP *Minicircle* Manufacturing

A prerequisite for clinical utilization of MCs in Germany and Europe is the ability of GMP manufacturing to satisfy regulatory requirements, even if the MC DNA is not directly injected in patients but rather used as a gene-transfer tool to modify T cells ex vivo as described here. Once their GMP manufacturing has been established, MCs will provide a tool that enables cost-effective, exportable manufacturing of CAR T cells, rapid evaluation of novel concepts in CAR T cell therapy in the academic setting, as well as scalable manufacture of validated CAR technologies for large patient cohorts to improve the outcome of prevalent hematologic and solid tumor malignancies.

Further, a process for *high-quality* grade MC production (Schmeer and Schleef 2014) will be established that will be used for subsequent viral vector or RNA production, since full GMP is often requested but in fact not necessary for these applications.

4.2 Clinical Implementation

As of July 2016, all clinical trials of CAR T cell therapy that reported clinical efficacy have used RV or LV to accomplish CAR gene-transfer (Maude et al. 2014; Davila et al. 2014; Turtle et al. 2016; Ramos et al. 2014). The results of clinical trials that employed CAR T cells that were generated by non-viral gene-transfer with SB transposition from conventional plasmids were rather disappointing; however, the lack of efficacy may have been caused by reasons related to the design of the specific CAR construct that was used in these trials and T cell composition of the CAR T cell products and be unrelated to the gene-transfer strategy that has been employed. It has been shown that CAR design and composition of CAR T cell products profoundly affect efficacy (Hudecek et al. 2013, 2015; Sommermeyer et al. 2016).

The use of non-viral gene-transfer and MCs to deliver SB transposase and CAR transposons into T cells is conceptually attractive and has significant potential to become the new gold standard in this field.

References

Aronovich EL, McIvor RS, Hackett PB (2011) The Sleeping Beauty transposon system: a non-viral vector for gene therapy. Hum Mol Genet 20(R1):R14–R20

Beatty GL, Haas AR, Maus MV et al (2014) Mesothelin-specific chimeric antigen receptor mRNA-engineered T cells induce anti-tumor activity in solid malignancies. Cancer Immunol Res. 2(2):112–120

Bigger BW, Tolmachov O, Collomber JM, Fragkos M, Palaszewski I, Coutelle C (2001) An araC-controlled bacterial cre expression system to produce DNA MC vectors for nuclear and mitochondrial gene therapy. J Biol Chem 276:23018–23027

Brentjens RJ, Riviere I, Park JH et al (2011) Safety and persistence of adoptively transferred autologous CD19-targeted T cells in patients with relapsed or chemotherapy refractory B-cell leukemias. Blood 118(18):4817–4828

Brown CE, Wright CL, Naranjo A et al (2005) Biophotonic cytotoxicity assay for high-throughput screening of cytolytic killing. J Immunol Methods 297(1–2):39–52

Chabot S, Orio J et al (2013) Minicircle DNA Electrotransfer for efficient Tissue targeted Gene Delivery. Gene Ther 20(1):62–68

Chen ZY, He CY, Ehrhardt A, Kay MA (2003) MC DNA vectors devoid of bacterial DNA result in persistent and high-level transgene expression in vivo. Mol Ther 8:495–500

Darquet AM, Cameron B, Wils P, Scherman D, Crouzet J (1997) A new DNA vehicle for nonviral gene delivery: supercoiled MC. Gene Ther 4:1341–1349

Davila ML, Riviere I, Wang X et al (2014) Efficacy and toxicity management of 19-28z CAR T cell therapy in B cell acute lymphoblastic leukemia. Sci Transl Med. 6(224):224–225

Di Stasi A, Tey SK, Dotti G et al (2011) Inducible apoptosis as a safety switch for adoptive cell therapy. N Engl J Med 365(18):1673–1683

Eberl L, Kristensen CS, Givskov M, Grohmann E, Gerlitz M, Schwab H (1994) Analysis of the multimer resolution system encoded by the *parCBA* operon of broad-host-range plasmid RP4. Mol Microbiol 12:131–141

Field AC, Vink C, Gabriel R et al (2013) Comparison of lentiviral and sleeping beauty mediated alphabeta T cell receptor gene-transfer. PLoS ONE 8(6):e68201

Gossen JA, de Leeuw WJF, Molijn AC et al (1993) Plasmid rescue from transgenic mouse DNA using lacI repressor protein conjugated to magnetic beads. Biotechniques 14:624–629

Huang X, Guo H, Kang J et al (2008) Sleeping Beauty transposon-mediated engineering of human primary T cells for therapy of CD19+ lymphoid malignancies. Mol Ther 16(3):580–589

Hudecek M, Lupo-Stanghellini MT, Kosasih PL et al (2013) Receptor affinity and extracellular domain modifications affect tumor recognition by ROR1-specific chimeric antigen receptor T cells. Clin Cancer Res 19(12):3153–3164

Hudecek M, Sommermeyer D, Kosasih PL et al (2015) The nonsignaling extracellular spacer domain of chimeric antigen receptors is decisive for in vivo antitumor activity. Cancer Immunol Res. 3(2):125–135

Ivics Z, Hackett PB, Plasterk RH, Izsvak Z (1997) Molecular reconstruction of Sleeping Beauty, a Tc1-like transposon from fish, and its transposition in human cells. Cell 91(4):501–510

Izsvak Z, Hackett PB, Cooper LJ, Ivics Z (2010) Translating Sleeping Beauty transposition into cellular therapies: victories and challenges. BioEssays 32(9):756–767

Ivics Z, Izsvak Z (2011) Nonviral gene delivery with the sleeping beauty transposon system. Hum Gene Ther 22(9):1043–1051

Jechlinger W, Azimpour Tabrizi T, Lubitz W, Mayrhofer P (2004) MC DNA immobilized in bacterial ghosts: in vivo production of safe non-viral DNA delivery vehicles. J Mol Microbiol Biotechnol 8:222–231

Jin Z, Maiti S, Huls H et al (2011) The hyperactive Sleeping Beauty transposase SB100X improves the genetic modification of T cells to express a chimeric antigen receptor. Gene Ther 18(9):849–856

Kolbelt D, Schleef M, Schmeer M, Aumann J, Schlag PM, Walther W (2013) Performance of high quality minicircle DNA for in vitro and in vivo gene-transfer. Mol Biotechnol 53(1):80–89

Mates L, Chuah MK, Belay E et al (2009) Molecular evolution of a novel hyperactive Sleeping Beauty transposase enables robust stable gene-transfer in vertebrates. Nat Genet 41(6):753–761

Maude SL, Frey N, Shaw PA et al (2014) Chimeric antigen receptor T cells for sustained remissions in leukemia. N Engl J Med 371(16):1507–1517

Mayrhofer P, Blaesen M, Schleef M, Jechlinger W (2008) Minicircle-DNA production by site specific recombination and protein-DNA interaction chromatography. J Gene Med 10(11):1253–1269

Monjezi R, Miskey C, Gogishvili T et al (2016) Enhanced CAR T-cell engineering using non-viral Sleeping Beauty transposition from minicircle vectors. Leukemia. doi:10.1038/leu.2016.180 (epub ahead of print)

Nehlsen K, Broll S, Bode J (2006) Replicating MCs: generation of nonviral episomes for the efficient modification of dividing cells. Gene Ther Mol Biol 10:233–244

Peng PD, Cohen CJ, Yang S et al (2009) Efficient nonviral Sleeping Beauty transposon-based TCR gene-transfer to peripheral blood lymphocytes confers antigen-specific antitumor reactivity. Gene Ther 16(8):1042–1049

Ramos CA, Savoldo B, Dotti G (2014) CD19-CAR trials. Cancer J 20(2):112–118

Sadelain M, Papapetrou EP, Bushman FD (2011) Safe harbours for the integration of new DNA in the human genome. Nat Rev Cancer 12(1):51–58

Schleef M, Schmeer M (2011) Minicircle—Die nächste Generation nicht-viraler Gentherapie-Vektoren. Parm unserer Zeit 3:220–224

Schleef M (ed) (2013) MC and Miniplasmid DNA vectors—the future of non-viral and viral gene-transfer. Wiley-Blackwell, Weinheim

Schleef M, Schirmbeck R, Reiser M, Michel M-L, Schmeer M (2015) MC: next generation DNA vectors for vaccination. In: Walther W, Stein U (eds) Gene therapy of solid cancers: methods and protocols (Methods in Molecular Biology) vol 1317. Springer, New York

Schmeer M, Schleef M (2014) Pharmaceutical grade large-scale plasmid DNA manufacturing process. In: Rinaldi M et al (eds) Methods in molecular biology, DNA Vaccines, vol 1143, pp 219–240. Springer, Heidelberg

Singh H, Manuri PR, Olivares S et al (2008) Redirecting specificity of T cell populations for CD19 using the Sleeping Beauty system. Cancer Res 68(8):2961–2971

Singh H, Figliola MJ, Dawson MJ et al (2013) Manufacture of clinical-grade CD19-specific T cells stably expressing chimeric antigen receptor using Sleeping Beauty system and artificial antigen presenting cells. PLoS ONE 8(5):e64138

Singh H, Huls H, Kebriaei P, Cooper LJ (2014) A new approach to gene therapy using Sleeping Beauty to genetically modify clinical-grade T cells to target CD19. Immunol Rev 257(1):181–190

Smith MC, Thorpe HM (2002) Diversity in the serine recombinases. Mol Microbiol 44:299–307

Sommermeyer D, Hudecek M, Kosasih PL et al (2016) Chimeric antigen receptor-modified T cells derived from defined CD8+ and CD4+ subsets confer superior antitumor reactivity in vivo. Leukemia 30(2):492–500

Swierczek M, Izsvak Z, Ivics Z (2012) The Sleeping Beauty transposon system for clinical applications. Expert Opin Biol Ther 12(2):139–153

Thomson JG, Ow DW (2006) Site-specific recombination systems for the genetic manipulation of eukaryotic genomes. Genesis 44:465–476

Turtle CJ, Hudecek M, Jensen MC, Riddell SR (2012) Engineered T cells for anti-cancer therapy. Curr Opin Immunol 24(5):633–639

Turtle CJ, Hanafi LA, Berger C et al (2016) CD19 CAR-T cells of defined CD4+: CD8+ composition in adult B cell ALL patients. J Clin Invest. 126(6):2123–2138

Wang X, Chang WC, Wong CW et al (2011) A transgene-encoded cell surface polypeptide for selection, in vivo tracking, and ablation of engineered cells. Blood 118(5):1255–1263

Noncoding RNA for Cancer Gene Therapy

Xiaomin Zhong, Dongmei Zhang, Minmin Xiong and Lin Zhang

Abstract

Gene therapy is a prospective strategy to modulate gene expression level in specific cells to treat human inherited diseases, cancers, and acquired disorders. A subset of noncoding RNAs, microRNAs (miRNAs) and small interference RNAs (siRNAs), compose an important class of widely used effectors for gene therapy, especially in cancer treatment. Functioning through the RNA interference (RNAi) mechanism, miRNA and siRNA show potent ability in silencing oncogenic factors for cancer gene therapy. For a better understanding of this field, we reviewed the mechanism and biological function, the principles of design and synthesis, and the delivery strategies of noncoding RNAs with clinical potentials in cancer gene therapy.

Keywords

Noncoding RNA · MicroRNA · Small interference RNA · RNA interference · Cancer · Gene therapy

X. Zhong (✉) · D. Zhang · L. Zhang
Department of Obstetrics and Gynecology, Perelman School of Medicine, University of Pennsylvania, Philadelphia, PA 19104, USA
e-mail: zhongxm23@mail.sysu.edu.cn

X. Zhong · M. Xiong
Center for Stem Cell Biology and Tissue Engineering, Department of Biology, Zhongshan School of Medicine, Sun Yat-Sen University, Guangzhou 510080, P.R. China

D. Zhang
State Key Laboratory of Biotherapy/Collaborative Innovation Center of Biotherapy, West China Hospital, Sichuan University, Chengdu 610041, P.R. China

W. Walther (ed.), *Current Strategies in Cancer Gene Therapy*,
Recent Results in Cancer Research 209, DOI 10.1007/978-3-319-42934-2_4

Abbreviations

miRNA	MicroRNA
siRNA	Small interference RNA
RNAi	RNA interference
Ago2	Argonaute 2
RISC	RNA-induced silencing complex
TRBP	TAR-RNA binding protein
PACT	Protein activator of PKR
shRNA	Short hairpin RNA
TRC	The RNAi Consortium
DOPC	1,2-dioleoyl-sn-glycero-3-phosphatidylcholine

1 Introduction

Gene therapy is a method of modulating gene expression level by introducing exogenous genetic materials into specific cells to treat human diseases including cancers. The most frequently used genetic material in gene therapy is DNA and RNA. DNA molecules used in gene therapy are usually disease-related genes (or gene fragments) to achieve gain-of-function effects, as well as antisense oligonucleotides for loss-of-function results (Zamecnik and Stephenson 1978). In the case of RNA, a subset of noncoding RNAs, microRNA (miRNA) and small interference RNA (siRNA), are emerging as popular effectors for gene therapy (Table 1). They are RNAs of small molecular weight, without protein-coding potentials. They have been shown to have potent biological functions accomplished by the mechanism of RNA interference (RNAi), which is a process triggered by double-stranded RNA molecules (Fire et al. 1998; Elbashir et al. 2001) and has been proved to be a powerful approach for reducing expression of mRNAs encoding pathogenic factors.

Table 1 Characteristics of noncoding RNAs for cancer gene therapy

	microRNA	siRNA	shRNA
Length	Primary (various), precursor (~70 nt), mature (18–25 nt)	~21 nt	25–27 nt
RNA structure	Primary (contains a hairpin), precursor (hairpin), mature (double-stranded)	Double-stranded	Hairpin
Targeting specificity	Intrinsically determined by seed sequence	Artificially designed	Artificially designed
Production	Chemical synthesis, viral expression, transgene expression	Chemical synthesis	Viral expression
Delivery method	Viral, non-viral and transgene	Non-viral vectors	Viral vectors

1.1 Mechanism and Function of Noncoding RNAs

miRNAs are endogenous small noncoding RNAs of ~18–25 nucleotides in length that regulate gene expression in a sequence-specific manner via the degradation of target mRNAs or the inhibition of protein translation. Most miRNA genes are transcribed by RNA Pol II to produce primary miRNA transcripts (pri-miRNAs) that contain a 5′ cap and a 3′ poly(A) tail (Lee et al. 2004; Cai et al. 2004). Pri-miRNAs harbor local hairpin structures and flanking sequences, which are subsequently cleaved within the nucleus by Drosha and DGCR8/Pasha (Denli et al. 2004; Gregory et al. 2004; Lee et al. 2003), to generate ~70-nt hairpin precursors known as pre-miRNAs. Next, the pre-miRNA is exported into the cytoplasm by Exportin-5 and further cleaved into a mature ~22-nt miRNA:miRNA* duplex by an RNase III enzyme Dicer, and its partners TRBP (TAR-RNA binding protein)/ Loquacious and PACT (protein activator of PKR) in human cells (Hutvagner et al. 2001; Ketting et al. 2001). Subsequently, an RNA-induced silencing complex called RISC is assembled with the protein Argonaute (Ago) 2 (Gregory et al. 2005; Maniataki and Mourelatos 2005). The miRNA strand is selectively incorporated into the RISC complex (Schwarz et al. 2003; Du and Zamore 2005) and guides the complex specifically to its mRNA targets through complementary base-pairing interactions between the seed sequence (base 2–8 in the 5′ end of the mature miRNA) and the binding site within target mRNAs. Through this mechanism, they exert their silencing functions by either mRNA degradation or translation inhibition (Fig. 1).

miRNAs exhibit a wide range of physiological functions, especially in cancer biology. Some miRNAs act as oncogenes or tumor suppressors. For example, oncogene miR-21 is upregulated in cancer cells, promotes cell growth, and suppresses apoptosis (Chan et al. 2005; Krichevsky and Gabriely 2009). Tumor suppressor let-7 family is usually downregulated or deleted in multiple cancer types, and restoration of let-7 expression leads to regression of tumors (Kumar et al. 2008; Johnson et al. 2007; Esquela-Kerscher et al. 2008; Takamizawa et al. 2004; Yang et al. 2008). miR-200 family is well known to be associated with cancer cell metastasis and apoptosis (Park et al. 2008; Gregory et al. 2008; Schickel et al. 2010). Based on the knowledge, efforts to overexpress tumor suppressor miRNAs and inhibit oncogene miRNAs to treat cancers have achieved positive results. Slack et al. delivered exogenous let-7 to established mouse models of non-small cell lung cancer and significantly reduces tumor burden (Trang et al. 2010). Naldini et al. functionally knocked down miR-223 expression by introducing decoy miRNA targets into mouse models (Gentner et al. 2009). Techniques for successful administration of miRNAs in vivo make it possible for miRNAs to act as good candidates for cancer therapy.

Much like miRNA, siRNA and shRNA are also potent mediators of sequence-specific gene silencing by RNAi mechanism. siRNA is a double-stranded small RNA of ~21 nt in length. It is exogenously synthesized as oligonucleotides (hereafter named as siRNA), or generated by 25–27-nt short hairpin RNA (shRNA) expressed from a DNA vector. The transcript of shRNA forms a stem-loop structure

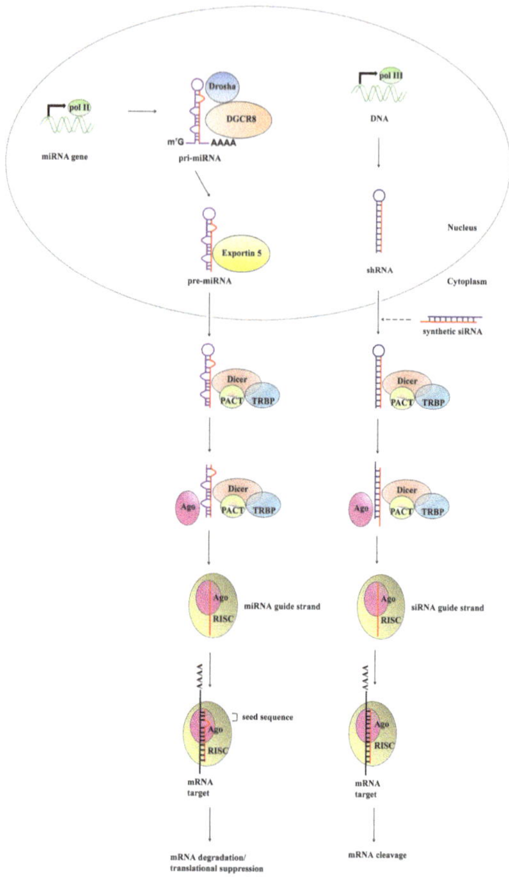

Fig. 1 The biogenesis process and RNAi mechanism of miRNA and siRNA/shRNA. Most miRNA genes are transcribed by RNA polymerase II (pol II) to produce primary miRNA transcripts (pri-miRNAs) that contain a 5′ cap and a 3′ poly(A) tail. Pri-miRNAs are subsequently cleaved within the nucleus by Drosha and DGCR8/Pasha to generate ~70-nt hairpin precursors known as pre-miRNAs. The pre-miRNA is exported into the cytoplasm by Exportin-5 and further cleaved into a mature ~22-nt miRNA:miRNA* duplex by Dicer, and its partners TRBP and PACT. Subsequently, an RNA-induced silencing complex called RISC is assembled with the protein Argonaute (Ago). The miRNA strand (guide strand) is selectively incorporated into the RISC complex and guides the complex to its mRNA targets through complementary base-pairing interactions between the seed sequence (base 2–8 in the 5′ end of the mature miRNA) and the binding site within target mRNAs. The target mRNA is silenced by either mRNA degradation or translation inhibition. Similarly, shRNA with stem-loop structure is transcribed by RNA polymerase III (pol III). In the cytoplasm, shRNA and synthetic siRNA are subject to the processing by Dicer and its partners TRBP and PACT to give rise to double-stranded ~21-nt siRNA. The guide strand of siRNA is assembled into RISC for target cleavage and gene silencing by RNAi mechanism. miRNA, microRNA; siRNA, small interference RNA; shRNA, short hairpin RNA; RISC, RNA-induced silencing complex

which can be further processed by Dicer to give rise to double-stranded ~21-nt siRNA. By either way, the functional guide strand of siRNA is assembled into RISC for target silencing by RNAi mechanism (Fig. 1). The interactions of siRNA and their targets are based on full complementarity of base pairing, which is different from miRNAs. The biological functions of siRNAs are mainly dependent on their target genes, because siRNAs can be flexibly designed and synthesized to target and modulate the function of any transcript theoretically. To date, siRNA has been extensively used in cancer gene therapy by targeting oncogenes such as *BCL-2* (in chronic myeloid leukemia), tyrosine kinase receptor *EphA2* gene (in ovarian cancer cells) (Landen et al. 2005), and *Ews–Fli1* gene fusion (in Ewing sarcoma cells) (Hu-Lieskovan et al. 2005).

1.2 Design and Synthesis of Noncoding RNAs for Cancer Gene Therapy

For gene therapy, the efficacy of exogenous genetic materials is largely determined by the compatibility with endogenous cellular machinery to perform their functions, as well as the delivery methods. However, multiple side effects of miRNA and siRNA in cancer gene therapy have been reported, including off-target effects, induction of immune system responses (Robbins et al. 2009), and saturation of endogenous RNAi pathway components (Khan et al. 2009; Grimm et al. 2006). The side effects sometimes can cause severe clinical outputs, thus limit the application of noncoding RNAs in gene therapy. To maximize the efficacy and minimize the side effects, it is necessary to follow some rules when designing noncoding RNAs for cancer gene therapy. Generally, it is important to consider the targeting sequences, the length, and the chemical modification of 3′ and 5′ ends of noncoding RNAs.

Synthetic miRNAs are usually present in the form of pri- or pre-miRNAs. Their targeting sequences (i.e., seed sequences) are determined by the nature of a specific miRNA. For synthetic siRNA and expressed shRNA, the targeting sequences are fully complementary to and determined by target mRNA sequences. The public TRC portal launched by the Broad Institute (The RNAi Consortium, http://www.broadinstitute.org/rnai/public/), as well as some commercial siRNA manufacturers, have developed online tools to help design specific and potent targeting sequences of siRNA based on the consideration of mRNA target sequence, secondary structures, siRNA stability, and minimizing sequence-dependent off-target effects. In addition, when designing targeting sequences for an interest gene, one should always pay attention to avoid the immunostimulatory effect of the synthetic sequences. It was reported that transfection of siRNA elicited interferon (IFN) responses (Sledz et al. 2003). A strategy to minimize this side effect is to avoid immunostimulatory sequences in siRNA design, e.g., 5′-GUCCUUCAA-3′ and 5′-UGUGU-3′ (Hornung et al. 2005; Judge et al. 2005).

In addition to the targeting sequence, the length and the modification of 3′ and 5′ ends of noncoding RNAs for cancer gene therapy also need to be paid attention to.

It was reported that 27-bp double-stranded RNAs can be up to 100 times more potent than 21-mer siRNAs due to more efficient processing by Dicer, and incorporation of DNA nucleotides into siRNA also enhanced Dicer processing (Kim et al. 2004, 2005). To reduce interferon production in target cells, avoiding 5′ triphosphates of siRNA by chemical synthesis needs to be considered (Kim et al. 2004). Similarly, 2-nt 3′ overhangs alleviate interferon induction effect by resembling endogenous products processed by Dicer (e.g., mature miRNA) (Marques et al. 2006). In addition, 2′-*O*-methyl modification of siRNA increases the stability and retains targeting specificity, but reduces interferon production (Judge et al. 2006; Morrissey et al. 2005). Conjugating cholesterol to the sense strand of the siRNA duplex is another common modification that manifested to be a successful strategy to enhance systemic delivery efficiency by promoting liver uptake of siRNA (Soutschek et al. 2004).

1.3 Delivery of Noncoding RNAs for Cancer Gene Therapy

Besides the chemical structures (RNA sequence and end modification), in vivo delivery method is another critical determinant affecting the efficacy of noncoding RNAs for cancer gene therapy. The obstacles for in vivo delivery include protecting from endogenous nuclease digestion, evading immune detection, and promoting extravasation from blood vessels to target tissues and cells. To overcome these obstacles, a variety of in vivo delivery methods for noncoding RNAs have been developed (Table 2).

Table 2 Delivery methods of noncoding RNAs for cancer gene therapy

Method	RNA species delivered	Advantages	Disadvantages
Non-viral vectors			
Naked delivery	miRNA, siRNA	No carriers needed	High dosage required
Lipid-based carriers	miRNA, siRNA	Robust, effective, and selective delivery	Sophisticated preparation needed
Polymersomes	siRNA	Robust, effective, and selective delivery	Sophisticated preparation needed
Cell-penetrating peptides	miRNA (e.g., pHLIP)	Effective and selective delivery	Expensive, sophisticated preparation
Inorganic nanoparticles	siRNA	Easy preparation	Limited efficiency, sometimes toxic
Viral vectors	miRNA, shRNA	Effective delivery, stable expression	Biosafety risk, immunogenic
Transgene	miRNA	Stable expression, non-immunogenic	Research purpose only

Noncoding RNA molecules could be simply delivered in a naked form at a relatively high dosage; for example, a dose of 50 mg/kg with the inhibitor of oncomir miR-10b (antagomiR-10b) was injected via tail vein, and it successfully suppressed the metastasis of mouse breast cancer by silencing endogenous miR-10b (Ma et al. 2010). To protect noncoding RNA from degradation and enhance the delivery efficiency, a variety of synthetic vectors have been developed, such as lipid-based carriers (Li and Szoka 2007), polymersomes (Lee et al. 2005), cell-penetrating peptides (Martin and Rice 2007), and inorganic nanoparticles (Sokolova and Epple 2008). Using nanoliposomes 1,2-dioleoyl-sn-glycero-3-phosphatidylcholine (DOPC), Calin et al. demonstrated successful delivery of both miR-520d-3p and *EphA2*-targeting siRNA to mouse model and found that the dual therapy was more potent in antitumor efficiency than either monotherapy alone due to simultaneously targeting both *EphA2* and *EphB2* oncogenes (Nishimura et al. 2013). Viral vectors are also widely used to express noncoding RNAs in vivo. Commonly used viral vectors for this purpose include retrovirus, lentivirus, adenovirus, and adeno-associated virus. Using an adeno-associated virus vector, systemic administration of miR-26a in a mouse model of liver cancer resulted in retarded growth and apoptosis induction of cancer cells (Kota et al. 2009). With an adenovirus vector, Slack and colleagues successfully delivered exogenous let-7 to established mouse models of non-small cell lung cancer and significantly reduces tumor burden (Trang et al. 2010). Naldini and colleagues presented technologies to functionally knock down miRNA expression by introducing decoy miRNA targets via lentiviral vectors into mouse models (Gentner et al. 2009). In addition, novel methods for in vivo delivery of noncoding RNAs are developing very fast. Recent study by Slack et al. reported that a novel construct, attachment of peptide nucleic acid anti-miRs to a peptide with a low pH-induced transmembrane structure (pHLIP), could transport an anti-miR-155 across plasma membranes under acidic conditions and reduced tumor growth. This method could selectively target the anti-miR to the acidic tumor microenvironment, evade systemic clearance by the liver, and facilitate cell entry via a non-endocytic pathway (Cheng et al. 2015). The discovery that a small molecule enoxacin (Penetrex) could enhance the activity of the RNAi pathway may also help to increase the efficacy of in vivo delivery of miRNA and siRNA (Shan et al. 2008).

For research purpose only, the technology of transgenic animal represents a liable method that is frequently employed to study in vivo function of expressed noncoding RNAs in cancer treatment. Inducible expression of miR-21 in a conditional transgenic mouse model revealed the oncogenic role of this miRNA in inducing pre-B-cell lymphoma and supports the efforts to treat human cancers through pharmacological inactivation of miRNAs such as miR-21 (Medina et al. 2010). The transgenic method provides valuable research data and applicable experience for related clinical trials.

2 Conclusion

miRNAs and siRNAs represent an extensively used class of noncoding effectors for cancer gene therapy. They both utilize RNAi mechanism to perform their biological functions in cancer treatment. The efficiency of miRNAs and siRNAs depends on multiple factors such as targeting sequence, end modification, and systemic delivery method. The understanding of the interaction between noncoding RNAs and their targets has been applied to clinical trials. To date, the targeting siRNAs for *BCL-2* (e.g., Chronic myeloid leukemia), *VEGF* (solid tumors), and *PLK1* (e.g., liver tumor) are undergoing or have completed clinical trials (from *ClinicalTrials.gov*). With progress in these studies, noncoding RNAs are believed to contribute a lot more to the field of cancer gene therapy.

Acknowledgments This work was supported, in whole or in part, by the Recruitment Project of Hundred Person of Sun Yat-Sen University (XZ), National Natural Science Foundation 81302262 (XZ), Guangdong Province Science and Technology Project 2015A020212019 (XZ), the Basser Research Center for BRCA (LZ), the National Institutes of Health R01CA142776 (LZ), R01CA190415 (LZ), P50CA083638 (LZ), P50CA174523 (LZ), the Breast Cancer Alliance (LZ), and the Marsha Rivkin Center for Ovarian Cancer Research (LZ).

References

Cai X, Hagedorn CH, Cullen BR (2004) Human microRNAs are processed from capped, polyadenylated transcripts that can also function as mRNAs. RNA 10(12):1957–1966
Chan JA, Krichevsky AM, Kosik KS (2005) MicroRNA-21 is an antiapoptotic factor in human glioblastoma cells. Cancer Res 65(14):6029–6033
Cheng CJ, Bahal R, Babar IA et al (2015) MicroRNA silencing for cancer therapy targeted to the tumour microenvironment. Nature 518(7537):107–110
Denli AM, Tops BB, Plasterk RH et al (2004) Processing of primary microRNAs by the Microprocessor complex. Nature 432(7014):231–235
Du T, Zamore PD (2005) microPrimer: the biogenesis and function of microRNA. Development 132(21):4645–4652
Elbashir SM, Harborth J, Lendeckel W et al (2001) Duplexes of 21-nucleotide RNAs mediate RNA interference in cultured mammalian cells. Nature 411(6836):494–498
Esquela-Kerscher A, Trang P, Wiggins JF et al (2008) The let-7 microRNA reduces tumor growth in mouse models of lung cancer. Cell Cycle 7(6):759–764
Fire A, Xu S, Montgomery MK et al (1998) Potent and specific genetic interference by double-stranded RNA in Caenorhabditis elegans. Nature 391(6669):806–811
Gentner B, Schira G, Giustacchini A et al (2009) Stable knockdown of microRNA in vivo by lentiviral vectors. Nat Methods 6(1):63–66
Gregory RI, Yan KP, Amuthan G et al (2004) The Microprocessor complex mediates the genesis of microRNAs. Nature 432(7014):235–240
Gregory RI, Chendrimada TP, Cooch N et al (2005) Human RISC couples microRNA biogenesis and posttranscriptional gene silencing. Cell 123(4):631–640
Gregory PA, Bert AG, Paterson EL et al (2008) The miR-200 family and miR-205 regulate epithelial to mesenchymal transition by targeting ZEB1 and SIP1. Nat Cell Biol 10(5):593–601
Grimm D, Streetz KL, Jopling CL et al (2006) Fatality in mice due to oversaturation of cellular microRNA/short hairpin RNA pathways. Nature 441(7092):537–541

Hornung V, Guenthner-Biller M, Bourquin C et al (2005) Sequence-specific potent induction of IFN-alpha by short interfering RNA in plasmacytoid dendritic cells through TLR7. Nat Med 11 (3):263–270

Hu-Lieskovan S, Heidel JD, Bartlett DW et al (2005) Sequence-specific knockdown of EWS-FLI1 by targeted, nonviral delivery of small interfering RNA inhibits tumor growth in a murine model of metastatic Ewing's sarcoma. Cancer Res 65(19):8984–8992

Hutvagner G, McLachlan J, Pasquinelli AE et al (2001) A cellular function for the RNA-interference enzyme Dicer in the maturation of the let-7 small temporal RNA. Science 293(5531):834–838

Johnson CD, Esquela-Kerscher A, Stefani G et al (2007) The let-7 microRNA represses cell proliferation pathways in human cells. Cancer Res 67(16):7713–7722

Judge AD, Sood V, Shaw JR et al (2005) Sequence-dependent stimulation of the mammalian innate immune response by synthetic siRNA. Nat Biotechnol 23(4):457–462

Judge AD, Bola G, Lee AC et al (2006) Design of noninflammatory synthetic siRNA mediating potent gene silencing in vivo. Mol Ther 13(3):494–505

Ketting RF, Fischer SE, Bernstein E et al (2001) Dicer functions in RNA interference and in synthesis of small RNA involved in developmental timing in *C. elegans*. Genes Dev 15 (20):2654–2659

Khan AA, Betel D, Miller ML et al (2009) Transfection of small RNAs globally perturbs gene regulation by endogenous microRNAs. Nat Biotechnol 27(6):549–555

Kim DH, Longo M, Han Y et al (2004) Interferon induction by siRNAs and ssRNAs synthesized by phage polymerase. Nat Biotechnol 22(3):321–325

Kim DH, Behlke MA, Rose SD et al (2005) Synthetic dsRNA Dicer substrates enhance RNAi potency and efficacy. Nat Biotechnol 23(2):222–226

Kota J, Chivukula RR, O'Donnell KA et al (2009) Therapeutic microRNA delivery suppresses tumorigenesis in a murine liver cancer model. Cell 137(6):1005–1017

Krichevsky AM, Gabriely G (2009) miR-21: a small multi-faceted RNA. J Cell Mol Med 13 (1):39–53

Kumar MS, Erkeland SJ, Pester RE et al (2008) Suppression of non-small cell lung tumor development by the let-7 microRNA family. Proc Natl Acad Sci U S A 105(10):3903–3908

Landen CN Jr, Chavez-Reyes A, Bucana C et al (2005) Therapeutic EphA2 gene targeting in vivo using neutral liposomal small interfering RNA delivery. Cancer Res 65(15):6910–6918

Lee Y, Ahn C, Han J et al (2003) The nuclear RNase III Drosha initiates microRNA processing. Nature 425(6956):415–419

Lee Y, Kim M, Han J et al (2004) MicroRNA genes are transcribed by RNA polymerase II. EMBO J 23(20):4051–4060

Lee CC, MacKay JA, Frechet JM et al (2005) Designing dendrimers for biological applications. Nat Biotechnol 23(12):1517–1526

Li W, Szoka FC Jr (2007) Lipid-based nanoparticles for nucleic acid delivery. Pharm Res 24 (3):438–449

Ma L, Reinhardt F, Pan E et al (2010) Therapeutic silencing of miR-10b inhibits metastasis in a mouse mammary tumor model. Nat Biotechnol 28(4):341–347

Maniataki E, Mourelatos Z (2005) A human, ATP-independent, RISC assembly machine fueled by pre-miRNA. Genes Dev 19(24):2979–2990

Marques JT, Devosse T, Wang D et al (2006) A structural basis for discriminating between self and nonself double-stranded RNAs in mammalian cells. Nat Biotechnol 24(5):559–565

Martin ME, Rice KG (2007) Peptide-guided gene delivery. AAPS J 9(1):E18–E29

Medina PP, Nolde M, Slack FJ (2010) OncomiR addiction in an in vivo model of microRNA-21-induced pre-B-cell lymphoma. Nature 467(7311):86–90

Morrissey DV, Lockridge JA, Shaw L et al (2005) Potent and persistent in vivo anti-HBV activity of chemically modified siRNAs. Nat Biotechnol 23(8):1002–1007

Nishimura M, Jung EJ, Shah MY et al (2013) Therapeutic synergy between microRNA and siRNA in ovarian cancer treatment. Cancer Discov 3(11):1302–1315

Park SM, Gaur AB, Lengyel E et al (2008) The miR-200 family determines the epithelial phenotype of cancer cells by targeting the E-cadherin repressors ZEB1 and ZEB2. Genes Dev 22(7):894–907

Robbins M, Judge A, MacLachlan I (2009) siRNA and innate immunity. Oligonucleotides 19 (2):89–102

Schickel R, Park SM, Murmann AE et al (2010) miR-200c regulates induction of apoptosis through CD95 by targeting FAP-1. Mol Cell 38(6):908–915

Schwarz DS, Hutvagner G, Du T et al (2003) Asymmetry in the assembly of the RNAi enzyme complex. Cell 115(2):199–208

Shan G, Li Y, Zhang J et al (2008) A small molecule enhances RNA interference and promotes microRNA processing. Nat Biotechnol 26(8):933–940

Sledz CA, Holko M, de Veer MJ et al (2003) Activation of the interferon system by short-interfering RNAs. Nat Cell Biol 5(9):834–839

Sokolova V, Epple M (2008) Inorganic nanoparticles as carriers of nucleic acids into cells. Angew Chem Int Ed Engl 47(8):1382–1395

Soutschek J, Akinc A, Bramlage B et al (2004) Therapeutic silencing of an endogenous gene by systemic administration of modified siRNAs. Nature 432(7014):173–178

Takamizawa J, Konishi H, Yanagisawa K et al (2004) Reduced expression of the let-7 microRNAs in human lung cancers in association with shortened postoperative survival. Cancer Res 64 (11):3753–3756

Trang P, Medina PP, Wiggins JF et al (2010) Regression of murine lung tumors by the let-7 microRNA. Oncogene 29(11):1580–1587

Yang N, Kaur S, Volinia S et al (2008) MicroRNA microarray identifies Let-7i as a novel biomarker and therapeutic target in human epithelial ovarian cancer. Cancer Res 68 (24):10307–10314

Zamecnik PC, Stephenson ML (1978) Inhibition of *Rous sarcoma* virus replication and cell transformation by a specific oligodeoxynucleotide. Proc Natl Acad Sci U S A 75(1):280–284

mRNA Cancer Vaccines

Katja Fiedler, Sandra Lazzaro, Johannes Lutz, Susanne Rauch and Regina Heidenreich

Abstract

mRNA cancer vaccines are a relatively new class of vaccines, which combine the potential of mRNA to encode for almost any protein with an excellent safety profile and a flexible production process. The most straightforward use of mRNA vaccines in oncologic settings is the immunization of patients with mRNA vaccines encoding tumor-associated antigens (TAAs). This is exemplified by the RNActive® technology, which induces balanced humoral and cellular immune responses in animal models and is currently evaluated in several clinical trials for oncologic indications. A second application of mRNA vaccines is the production of personalized vaccines. This is possible because mRNA vaccines are produced by a generic process, which can be used to quickly produce mRNA vaccines targeting patient-specific neoantigens that are identified by analyzing the tumor exome. Apart from being used directly to vaccinate patients, mRNAs can also be used in cellular therapies to transfect patient-derived cells in vitro and infuse the manipulated cells back into the patient. One such application is the transfection of patient-derived dendritic cells (DCs) with mRNAs encoding TAAs, which leads to the presentation of TAA-derived peptides on the DCs and an activation of antigen-specific T cells in vivo. A second application is the transfection of patient-derived T cells with mRNAs encoding chimeric antigen receptors, which allows the T cells to directly recognize a specific antigen expressed on the tumor. In this chapter, we will review preclinical and clinical data for the different approaches.

Keywords

RNActive® vaccines · Personalized mRNA vaccines · mRNA-pulsed dendritic cells · Chimeric antigen receptor (CAR) T cell immunotherapy

K. Fiedler (✉) · S. Lazzaro · J. Lutz · S. Rauch · R. Heidenreich
CureVac AG, Paul-Ehrlich-Str. 15, 72076 Tübingen, Germany
e-mail: katja.fiedler@curevac.com

W. Walther (ed.), *Current Strategies in Cancer Gene Therapy*,
Recent Results in Cancer Research 209, DOI 10.1007/978-3-319-42934-2_5

Abbreviations

A	Adenine
APC	Antigen-presenting cell
CAR	Chimeric antigen receptor
CTL	Cytotoxic T lymphocyte
CTLA4	Cytotoxic T lymphocyte antigen 4
DC	Dendritic cell
DNA	Deoxyribonucleic acid
EGFR	Endothelial growth factor receptor
ELISA	Enzyme-linked immunosorbent assay
GC	Guanine and cytosine
GITR	Glucocorticoid-induced tumor necrosis factor receptor
HLA	Human leukocyte antigen
HMGB1	High-mobility group box 1
IDH1	Isocitrate dehydrogenase 1
IFN	Interferon
Ig	Immunoglobulin
LLC	Lewis lung cancer
MAGEC1	Melanoma antigen family C1
MAGEC2	Melanoma antigen family C2
MHC	Major histocompatibility complex
mRNA	Messenger ribonucleic acid
MUC1	Mucin 1
NK	Natural killer
NSCLC	Non-small-cell lung cancer
NY-ESO-1	New York esophageal squamous cell carcinoma-1
ORF	Open reading frame
OVA	Ovalbumin
PAP	Prostatic acid phosphatase
PD1	Programmed cell death 1
PDL1	Programmed cell death 1 ligand 1
PDL2	Programmed cell death 1 ligand 2
PFS	Progression-free survival
PSA	Prostate-specific antigen
PSCA	Prostate stem cell antigen
PSMA	Prostate-specific membrane antigen
RNA	Ribonucleic acid
RT-PCR	Reverse transcriptase polymerase chain reaction
STEAP1	Six-transmembrane epithelial antigen of the prostate 1
TAA	Tumor-associated antigen
TERT	Telomerase reverse transcriptase
Th	T helper
TLR	Toll-like receptor

Tmeso	CAR T cells specifically targeting mesothelin
TPBG	Trophoblast glycoprotein
UTR	Untranslated region

1 mRNA Cancer Vaccines

1.1 Introduction

The concept of mRNA vaccines is founded on the observation that injection of messenger RNA (mRNA) leads to local protein expression (Wolff et al. 1990) and immune responses against the encoded antigen (Martinon et al. 1993). This was rather unexpected given the abundant presence of RNases in body fluids and on the skin, which leads to the rapid degradation of RNA, for example, in serum-containing media (Rammensee 2006), and most work on nucleic acid-based vaccine development continued to focus on DNA rather than on RNA vaccines. This view has changed with the advent of several technological platforms, which have demonstrated the potential of mRNA vaccines to express antigen and to induce humoral and cellular immune responses.

While both nucleic acid-based platforms share many characteristics, mRNA vaccines have several advantages over DNA-based platforms (Table 1). Firstly, RNA only needs to pass the plasma membrane in order to induce protein synthesis, facilitating vaccine delivery in comparison with DNA that needs to additionally cross the nuclear membrane. Secondly, mRNA is unable to integrate in the genome and therefore has no oncogenic potential. Finally, expression of mRNA-encoded proteins is intrinsically transient, defined by the short half-life of mRNA. Hence, mRNA vaccines feature a significantly increased safety profile over DNA.

In addition, mRNA vaccines provide important advantages over the more widely used protein-based vaccine platforms: Endogenous production of proteins in the cells of the vaccinee upon injection of mRNA supports correct protein modifications, such as glycosylation patterns, and abolishes the need for elaborate protein or particle purification steps. From a technical perspective, mRNA, unlike protein-based vaccines, can be produced in a fully synthetic production process and allows the production of mRNA encoding any protein or combination of proteins of choice using the same biologic compounds and production steps, greatly facilitating vaccine manufacturing processes. Furthermore, the ability to support quick sequence adjustments makes RNA vaccines highly versatile, which is of particular importance in pandemic settings or for individualized therapies (see below).

1.2 RNActive® Vaccines

The first section focuses on the RNActive® technology (CureVac AG), as an example for an mRNA vaccine platform currently evaluated in several clinical trials for oncologic indications.

RNActive® vaccines consist of formulated mRNA which encodes for the antigenic protein of choice and features modifications to enhance translation efficiency, delay mRNA decay, and improve immune stimulation.

In 2000, Hoerr et al. described that the in vivo application of mRNA encoding the model antigen β-galactosidase led to the induction of specific cytotoxic T lymphocytes (CTLs) and antibodies (Hoerr et al. 2000). The RNA used for these experiments had the basic design of a mRNA and consisted of a cap, an open reading frame (ORF) encoding for β-galactosidase that was flanked 5′ and 3′ by the untranslated regions (UTRs) of β-globin and a poly(A) tail. For the current RNActive® technology, several aspects of the mRNAs have been modified to increase the extent and duration of the antigen expression. The β-globin UTRs have been replaced by UTRs selected for higher translation efficiency and stability of the mRNAs, and the ORF was optimized for enhanced protein expression by enriching the guanine and cytosine (GC) content according to a proprietary algorithm. These changes, as well as the use of a template-encoded poly(A) tail of defined length, optimized buffers, and purification led to an increase in protein expression by four to five orders of magnitude in various test systems (Kallen and Theß 2014). Importantly, this technology exclusively employs unmodified nucleotides. Studies by Karikó (Karikó et al. 2008) and Anderson (Anderson et al. 2010) have demonstrated that modified nucleotides can lead to increased protein expression. However, they also reduced immunogenicity, making the use of modified nucleotides unfavorable in the context of vaccines.

In addition to antigen availability, adjuvanticity is essential for inducing strong immune responses. In RNActive® vaccines, immunostimulatory capacity is achieved via suitable formulation, e.g., by employing protamine, a cationic peptide that forms stable complexes with nucleic acids. Protamine binds to the mRNA and leads to the formation of larger particles that activate the immune system in a process involving the endosome-resident TLR7 (Toll-like receptor 7) (Fotin-Mleczek et al. 2011; Kallen et al. 2013; Scheel et al. 2005; Kowalczyk et al. 2016) (Table 1).

Hence, RNActive® vaccines are containing two components that serve complementary functions: “naked” mRNA, which serves as a translation template responsible for strong expression of the encoded antigen, and mRNA–protamine complexes, which enhance the immune stimulatory capacity of the vaccine. Indeed, vaccination with RNActive® vaccines has been shown to induce strong and balanced immune responses, i.e., Th1 and Th2, humoral and cellular, and effector and memory responses. Encouraging results have been gained in various animal model systems, among others mice, ferrets, and pigs, both in the field of cancer

Table 1 Advantages of RNA over DNA vaccines

	DNA	RNA
Delivery	DNA needs to cross both cell and nuclear membranes and be first transcribed in the nucleus before protein expression occurs	RNA only needs to gain entry into the cytoplasm, where translation and thus protein expression directly occur
Integration	DNA vaccines are able to integrate into the host genome, which might result in insertional mutagenesis and chromosomal instability	RNA cannot integrate into the genome and therefore has no oncogenic potential
Expression	Long-term expression possible (months to years), depending on vector	Transient expression

immunotherapy (Fotin-Mleczek et al. 2011, 2012) and prophylactic vaccines (Petsch et al. 2012; Kowalczyk et al. 2016; Schnee et al. 2016).

1.2.1 Induction of Antitumor Responses with RNActive® Vaccines

The antitumor efficacy of RNActive® vaccines was initially studied in the E. G7-OVA tumor model. This system uses C57BL/6 mice, which are inoculated subcutaneously with the syngeneic E.G7-OVA cell line, a clone of the mouse thymoma EL4 cell line that has been stably transfected to express ovalbumin (Moore et al. 1988). The vaccine was first studied in a prophylactic setting. Mice were immunized twice intradermally with the mRNA vaccine encoding ovalbumin and challenged one week later with E.G7-OVA cells. Compared to control mice that had received an mRNA vaccine encoding for an irrelevant antigen, the OVA-RNActive®-treated group displayed a significant delay in tumor growth (Fotin-Mleczek et al. 2011). Additionally, vaccination with OVA-RNActive® induced superior tumor protection in comparison with vaccination with ovalbumin protein or OVA-peptide SIINFEKL (Fotin-Mleczek et al. 2012).

A detailed analysis revealed that the antigen-specific vaccination had induced a balanced humoral and cellular immune responses with high titers of ovalbumin-specific IgG1 and IgG2a antibodies and cytotoxic T cells, which secreted IFN-γ upon stimulation with an OVA-derived peptide in vitro and killed OVA-peptide-loaded cells in vivo. Further experiments employing the antigen PSMA showed that the cytotoxic response was boostable and led to the formation of T memory cells. Increasing the number of biweekly vaccinations with the PSMA-RNActive® vaccine from 2 to 4 or 6 vaccinations induced a significant increase in both number of IFN-γ-secreting $CD8^+$ T cells and in vivo cytotoxicity during the acute phase. When analyzing these mice in the memory phase 8 weeks after the last immunization, a similar increase in the number of IFN-γ-secreting $CD8^+$ T cells and in vivo cytotoxicity was observed by increasing the number of vaccinations. Importantly, these IFN-γ-secreting $CD8^+$ T cells displayed the memory T cell marker CD44 and predominantly exhibited an effector memory phenotype ($CD44^+$, $CCR7^-$, $CD62L^-$). Moreover, repeated vaccinations did not induce detectable frequencies of regulatory T cells in mice in comparison with controls (Fotin-Mleczek et al. 2011).

To test the efficacy of this technology in a therapeutic setting, the E.G7-OVA model was again employed. Mice were challenged subcutaneously with the tumor cells and received the OVA-RNActive® vaccine twice a week once the tumor was palpable. The treatment led to a significant delay in tumor growth but could not eradicate the tumor. A subsequent quantitative RT-PCR analysis showed that the ovalbumin expression in the outgrown tumors of all mice treated with the ovalbumin-encoding mRNA vaccine was reduced or even absent, while this was only the case in 1/5 of the untreated mice. This indicates that the tumors in RNActive® vaccine-treated mice had escaped immunotherapy due to downregulation of ovalbumin (Fotin-Mleczek et al. 2011).

Analysis of the cellular composition of tumors at several time points after vaccination demonstrated an increased and sustained influx of activated $CD8^+$ T cells into the tumors in vaccinated mice. Depletion of $CD8^+$ T cells, but not of $CD4^+$ T cells, during the effector phase completely abolished the antitumor effect of the vaccine. In contrast, $CD4^+$ T cells are required during the priming phase of the immune response as their depletion during vaccination significantly reduced vaccine efficacy (Fotin-Mleczek et al. 2011).

1.2.2 Clinical Studies with RNActive® Vaccines

Based on the encouraging preclinical results, the decision was taken to advance this technology to clinical testing in cancer patients (Table 2). The first-in-class first-in-man clinical trial using mRNA as a therapeutic approach was CV9103 for patients with prostate cancer. CV9103 is an RNActive® vaccine targeting the following 4 tumor-associated antigens: prostate-specific antigen (PSA), prostate-specific membrane antigen (PSMA), prostate stem cell antigen (PSCA), and six-transmembrane epithelial antigen of the prostate 1 (STEAP1). The vaccine was tested in a phase I/IIa study that enrolled 44 eligible patients with castrate-resistant prostate cancer with rising levels of PSA (all patients) and metastatic disease in 84 % of patients and comprised 12 men in the phase I and 32 in the phase IIa study (Kübler et al. 2015). The study was conducted as an open, uncontrolled, multicenter, international, and prospective trial with safety and tolerability defined as the primary endpoints and the induction of antigen-specific humoral and cellular immune responses as secondary endpoints. The recommended dose was established via a dose escalation in the phase I trial (259, 640, and 1280 µg total RNA tested), while the phase IIa study was designed to confirm safety and address the induction of antigen-specific cellular and humoral immune responses following injection with the highest dose. This study demonstrated that CV9103 exhibits a favorable safety profile with most frequent adverse events being injection site reactions, fatigue, pyrexia, chills, and flulike symptoms. The majority of related adverse events was of mild-to-moderate intensity and resolved upon therapy.

Importantly, immune responses against all mRNA-encoded antigens were detectable independent of the cellular localization of the antigen and the HLA

Table 2 Overview of clinical trials using RNActive® vaccines

Biologic	Indication	Phase	Antigens	*n*	Outcome	Reference
CV9103	Hormone refractory prostate cancer	I/IIa	PSA PSMA PSCA STEAP1	44	– Favorable safety profile – Induction of multiple antigen-specific immune responses – Induction of immune responses against all encoded antigens	Kübler et al. (2015)
CV9104	Metastatic castrate-refractory prostate cancer Asymptomatic, minimally symptomatic, chemonaive	I/IIb	MUC1 PAP PSA PSMA PSCA STEAP1	Ph IIb 197	Double-blind placebo-controlled study Recruitment completed	
CV9104	Intermediate- or high-risk prostate cancer prior to radical prostatectomy	II	MUC1 PAP PSA PSMA PSCA STEAP1	48	Open-label randomized trial of presurgical CV9104 vs no treatment Recruitment completed	
CV9201	Advanced-stage non-small-cell lung cancer	I/IIa	MAGEC1 MAGEC2 NY-ESO-1 Survivin 5T4	46	– Favorable safety profile – Induction of multiple antigen-specific immune responses – Induction of immune responses against all encoded antigens	Sebastian et al., manuscript in preparation
CV9202+ local radiation	Advanced-stage non-small-cell lung cancer	Ib	MAGEC1 MAGEC2 MUC1 NY-ESO-1 Survivin 5T4	26	Study ongoing	

subtype of the patient. More specifically, antigen-specific cellular immune responses were detected in 76 % of all patients treated with the highest dose. Of note, 58 % of responding patients and 45 % of all evaluable patients at the highest dose level showed responses to multiple antigens. The assessment of humoral immune responses was restricted to PSA and PSCA, since no proteins suitable for ELISA were available for the other vaccination antigens at that time. An increase of PSA-specific antibodies could be detected in 12 % of patients, but no increase of anti-PSCA antibodies was observed.

Clinical efficacy of CV9103 was assessed mainly by progression of PSA serum levels, since radiographic progression-free survival (PFS) was not assessed in this clinical trial. Similar to other cancer vaccine trials, a median time to PSA-related PFS is 1.8 months and an objective PSA response in only one patient was observed.

Additionally, the study estimated a median survival of 31.4 months for a subgroup of 36 patients with metastatic castrate-resistant prostate cancer. In this group, a non-significant correlation between survival time and multivalent immune response was observed. Interestingly, outcome further improved in patients with responses to multiple vaccination antigens. Yet a correlation between immune responses against more than one antigen and improved survival time does not necessarily imply a therapeutic effect of vaccination. The ability to mount an immune response after vaccination might be instead a surrogate of an improved prognosis (Kübler et al. 2015).

Nevertheless, these encouraging results justified the investigation of RNActive® vaccines in a controlled clinical trial. Hence, 197 patients with castrate-resistant asymptomatic to minimally symptomatic castration-resistant prostate cancer were enrolled and randomized in an ongoing placebo-controlled phase IIb study with CV9104. This updated vaccine is based on CV9103 and encodes two additional tumor-associated antigens, namely prostatic acid phosphatase (PAP) and mucin 1 (MUC1), a glycoprotein that is overexpressed and aberrantly glycosylated in various cancers including prostate cancer. The clinical efficacy and safety of PAP as vaccine antigen have previously been demonstrated in the clinical trial of Sipuleucel-T (Kantoff et al. 2010), while MUC1 has mainly been used in immunotherapy approaches against non-small-cell lung cancer with a favorable safety profile (Palmer et al. 2001). Primary endpoint of the study is overall survival from time of randomization (up to 3.5–4 years). Secondary endpoints include PFS from date of randomization and from start of first subsequent systemic therapy, respectively, immune response against the CV9104 antigens, time to symptom progression, and change in quality of life.

In a second study, CV9104 is tested in patients with high- and intermediate-risk non-metastatic prostate cancer. For these patients, radical prostatectomy is a standard treatment option. After surgery, the estimated risk of relapse is considerable, even more in case of positive surgical margins. Hence, new adjuvant or neoadjuvant treatments that can prevent relapses after primary therapy are highly needed.

The study is aimed to assess the immune responses in the peripheral blood as well as immunological parameters in the tumor tissue such as cellular immune infiltrates, cytokines, and gene expression upon application of CV9104.

In addition to its application in the treatment of prostate cancer, RNActive® vaccines were also tested as an immunotherapeutic against non-small-cell lung carcinoma (NSCLC) in a clinical phase I/IIa trial (Sebastian et al., manuscript in preparation).

In this study, the immunotherapeutic CV9201 was intradermally administered at different dose levels to evaluate the safety and tolerability in patients with advanced NSCLC. CV9201 encodes five NSCLC-associated cancer antigens selected for their role in NSCLC oncogenesis, differential expression between malignant and normal tissue and to induce cellular or humoral immune responses: New York esophageal squamous cell carcinoma-1 (NY-ESO-1), melanoma antigen family C1 (MAGEC1), melanoma antigen family C2 (MAGEC2), survivin, and trophoblast glycoprotein (TPBG; synonym 5T4). Eligible patients had stage IIIB/IV NSCLC and at least stable disease after first-line treatment. During the open, uncontrolled, multicenter, and prospective trial, 9 patients received CV9201 in the phase I and 37 patients in the phase IIa part of the study. Overall, 45/46 patients received at least two treatments and 33/46 patients received all five planned doses of CV9201. This study demonstrated that similar to CV9103, also CV9201 exhibits a favorable safety profile with most frequent adverse events being injection site reactions, including injection site erythema, pruritus, discoloration, and pain. Other treatment-related adverse events were pyrexia and fatigue, chills, and flulike symptoms. Furthermore, immune responses against all encoded antigens were detectable. In detail, 65 % of all patients exhibited antigen-specific cellular or humoral immune responses and 65 % of responders reacted against multiple antigens. The strength of the induced T cell response varied, but most patients displayed a more-than-twofold increase in frequency and number of antigen-specific T cells detected ex vivo, with some patients showing very strong responses. Moreover, 48 % of the patients treated in phase IIa had antigen-specific humoral responses, with more than twice as many patients exhibiting IgM than IgG responses.

Tumor response was evaluable in 29 patients of which nine patients had stable disease and twenty patients experienced progressive disease as best overall response. The median PFS in the total study population was 2.7 months. Importantly, the study revealed an encouraging clinical course in five patients with stage IV NSCLC being without further systemic cancer therapy after 1 year.

Overall, these results demonstrate that RNActive® vaccines represent a highly promising new vaccine platform that is safe, highly specific, versatile, and able to induce a balance immune response in the context of clinical studies.

1.2.3 Combination of RNActive® Vaccines with Chemotherapy or Radiation Therapy

From a clinical perspective, it is important to assess whether RNActive® vaccines can be combined with the current standard of care. Therefore, the combination of these vaccines with chemotherapy or radiation therapy was investigated.

The combination with chemotherapy was tested in the E.G7-OVA tumor model using docetaxel or cisplatin and the mRNA vaccine against ovalbumin.

Having received a subcutaneous tumor challenge followed by RNActive® vaccinations, mice were subsequently treated with an intraperitoneal application of docetaxel followed by further vaccinations. This treatment schedule led to a significant delay in tumor growth compared to docetaxel or RNActive® vaccine alone. Similar results were observed when using the same treatment schedule but cisplatin as a chemotherapeutic drug. In agreement with published results using viral vector vaccines (Garnett et al. 2008), a delay of tumor growth was not detectable when chemotherapy preceded vaccination, indicating a negative effect of docetaxel during the induction phase of the immune response (Fotin-Mleczek et al. 2012).

An interesting option is the combination of vaccination with radiation therapy because of the complementary features of the two approaches, which can synergize to restrict tumor growth. Radiation is a well-established therapeutic method, especially for the treatment of single solid tumors. It acts on the tumor tissue locally and, for a very short period of time, is effective on tumors with a local immunosuppressive environment due to increased release of proinflammatory cytokines (Formenti and Demaria 2013) and induces local MHC expression (Reits et al. 2006). Moreover, radiotherapy-induced cell death seems to represent a form of immunogenic cell death characterized by cell surface translocation of calreticulin and extracellular release of ATP and the high-mobility group box 1 (HMGB1) protein (Golden et al. 2014). These factors are able to activate dendritic cells (DCs) via pattern recognition receptors and promote the cross-presentation of tumor antigens between DCs and T cells (Demaria and Formenti 2012).

Vaccination, on the other hand, is able to induce systemic immune responses against non-symptomatic metastatic disease that are long-lasting and boostable.

Hence, the combination of radiotherapy and RNActive® vaccines was tested in an E.G7-OVA tumor model. After the establishment of large subcutaneous tumors, the mice received three local radiations on consecutive days. Concomitantly, several vaccinations with OVA-RNActive® vaccine were administered. These experiments demonstrated a pronounced tumor regression in the group treated with combination therapy and complete eradication of large established E.G7-OVA tumors in 3 out of 7 mice, while single therapies remained significantly less effective (Fotin-Mleczek et al. 2014). Additional experiments were performed in the Lewis lung cancer (LLC) model as a second tumor system, which features low immunogenicity and is resistant to different kinds of therapeutic regimens (Savai et al. 2007; Shojaei et al. 2007; Knapp et al. 2003). After subcutaneous tumor challenge, the mice were treated with three local radiations on consecutive days in combination with several vaccinations with RNActive® vaccines encoding the described tumor-associated antigens EGFR and connexin (Mandelboim et al. 1995). The combined treatment showed a synergistic antitumor effect demonstrating the efficacy of radioimmunotherapy even in a low immunogenic carcinoma model system (Fotin-Mleczek et al. 2014).

1.2.4 Clinical Study with RNActive® Vaccines in Combination with Radiotherapy

Based on the promising preclinical results, a phase Ib study is ongoing, evaluating the clinical potential of the RNActive® vaccine CV9202 in combination with local radiation of individual metastases as consolidation and maintenance treatment for patients with stage IV non-small-cell lung cancer. CV9202 is an updated version of CV9201 that encodes in addition to NY-ESO-1, MAGEC1, MAGEC2, survivin, and 5T4, the antigen MUC1. As described earlier, the glycoprotein MUC1—overexpressed and aberrantly glycosylated in various cancers—has previously been used in immunotherapy approaches against non-small-cell lung cancer (Palmer et al. 2001). The exploratory, open-label multicenter trial assesses the safety and tolerability of CV9202 vaccination combined with local radiation in patients with stage IV NSCLC of different subtypes (squamous and non-squamous cell with or without EGFR mutations) who achieved a response or stable disease after first-line therapy (chemotherapy or EGFR tyrosine kinase inhibitors). All patients receive two initial vaccinations with CV9202 prior to local radiotherapy followed by further vaccinations until disease progression. The primary endpoint of the study is the number of patients experiencing treatment-related adverse events above grade 3. Secondary endpoints include evaluation of cellular and humoral immune responses to antigens encoded by CV9202 and antigens not covered by the vaccine allowing the investigation of potential antigen spreading in response to the treatment. In addition, assessment of PFS, time to start of second-line cancer treatment, response to second-line treatment, and overall survival are secondary efficacy endpoints of the study (Sebastian et al. 2014).

1.2.5 Combination of RNActive® Vaccines with Immune Checkpoint Inhibitors

The immune response to cancer evolves over many years and ultimately fails due to immunoediting (downregulation of MHC I and immunogenic antigens) and immunoevasion (immunosuppressive microenvironment) (Vesely and Schreiber 2013). Moreover, the antitumor immune response has many characteristics of a chronic immune response, with T cell exhaustion mediated by immune checkpoint receptors such as programmed cell death 1 (PD1). PD1 is also expressed by B cells, NK cells, and regulatory T cells in addition to activated T cells and is engaged by two different ligands PDL1 (B7-H1) and PDL2 (B7-DC). In contrast, the immune checkpoint receptor cytotoxic T lymphocyte antigen 4 (CTLA4) is only expressed by activated T cells or regulatory T cells, and binding of its ligands CD80 (B7-1) or CD86 (B7-2) leads to inhibition of T cells by antagonizing the costimulatory signals delivered by CD28 during T cell activation (Melero et al. 2015).

Various antibodies targeting these immune checkpoints are currently in clinical testing and show promising results for some of the patients. But there are still a substantial proportion of patients not reacting to immune checkpoint blockade. Newly published studies imply a strong correlation between the occurrence of antigen-specific T cells and response to immune checkpoint blockade (reviewed in Schumacher and Schreiber 2015). Hence, the induction of antigen-specific cellular response against tumor-associated antigens by vaccination would be beneficial during immune checkpoint blockade therapy. To test whether checkpoint inhibitors can also be combined with mRNA vaccines, an RNActive® vaccine was combined with an anti-CTLA-4 antibody. Mice were challenged with E.G7-OVA tumors and treated alternatingly with an ovalbumin-encoding mRNA vaccine and an anti-CTLA-4 antibody. The combination led to significantly reduced tumor growth, while anti-CTLA-4 treatment alone did not delay tumor growth. In addition, mice in which treatment had led to complete rejection were rechallenged with the parental tumor cell line, which lacks OVA expression. These experiments showed that the mice were nonetheless completely protected, strongly indicative of the induction of epitope spreading (Fotin-Mleczek et al. 2012).

In summary, the superior antitumor response of RNActive® vaccine treatment in combination with immune checkpoint blockade could be demonstrated in a pre-clinical animal model.

1.3 Personalized mRNA Vaccines

In the past, development of cancer vaccines was mainly dedicated toward the so-called tumor-associated proteins as antigenic source. Mostly, these tumor-associated antigens can be divided into two classes: Antigens derived from fetal genes overexpressed in cancer cells (van der Bruggen et al. 1991; Van den Eynde et al. 1991) or antigens derived from tissue-specific proteins also expressed in cancer cells (Boon et al. 1994). To offer broadly applicable immune therapies against cancer, the latest developmental activity in the field of cancer vaccines was focused on shared tumor-associated antigens that are expressed not only in abundance in different cancer types but also in a certain amount of cancer patients.

But the use of such shared tumor-associated antigens is accompanied with certain drawbacks: Firstly, T cells easily recognize foreign antigens but in general are unable to recognize self-antigens due to the negative selection process in the thymus preventing induction of autoimmunity. Unfortunately, most tumor-associated antigens fall into the group of self-antigens hampering the initiation of a proper immune response toward these antigens. Secondly, tumor-associated antigens are not solitarily expressed in tumor tissue leading to possible on-target effects in healthy tissue through the induced immune response. Finally, the expression of tumor-associated antigens in different tumor tissues or different cancer patients can be highly variable due to normal biologic heterogeneity. Recent research has shown that ninety-five percent of the mutations in a given patient seem to be unique to that tumor (Stratton 2011) and that even on a subclonal level a high variability can be found in a certain tumor (Gerlinger et al. 2015; Martincorena et al. 2015). Therefore, it can be assumed that expression of shared tumor-associated antigens is subjected to a similar variability. Moreover, tumor tissues often exploit different escape mechanisms to evade the antitumoral immune response like downregulation of tumor-associated antigens or preferential outgrowth of non-expressing clones (Matsushita et al. 2012).

The use of really tumor-specific antigens or neoantigens instead of tumor-associated antigens would be advantageous for the development of cancer vaccines for obvious reasons: Owed to the tumor-specific mutations of these neoantigens, the specific T cell repertoire is not affected by negative selection in the thymus. In addition, neoantigen-specific T cells would not cause on-target effects on healthy tissue as mutated antigens are only expressed in cancer cells. Already in the 1970s and 1980s, the tumor-rejecting abilities of neoantigen-induced immune responses were described in transplantable tumor models (Boon and Kellermann 1977; Lurquin et al. 1989). Moreover, different studies could show that single mutations in defined genes are able to induce antigen-specific cytolytic T cell responses (Wölfel et al. 1995; Coulie et al. 1995; Echchakir et al. 2001).

The advent of next-generation sequencing technologies over the last years allows nowadays the definition of such tumor-specific antigens or neoantigens by comparing genome, exome, or transcriptome data of tumor tissue to healthy tissue for an individual patient. This approach allows the description of non-synonymous mutations solely expressed in tumor cells. Moreover, exome or transcriptome analysis permits the definition of protein abundance for defined non-synonymous mutations in the tumor tissue. This conglomerate of tumor-specific mutations, also named "mutanome," displayed by an individual tumor is a valuable source for highly tumor-specific antigens.

Two studies in mice provided the first direct evidence that neoantigens identified by mutanome analysis can be recognized by T cells (Castle et al. 2012; Matsushita et al. 2012). Briefly, potential MHC-binding peptides were predicted for all tumor-specific mutations that result in the formation of novel protein sequences and the most promising mutated peptides were used to query T cell reactivity in vivo. Castle and colleagues could show that 16 out of 50 mutation-coding peptides elicit a measurable immune response in immunized mice. Moreover, the induced immune response conferred a significant antitumor effect in a B16F10 tumor model. In the study of Matsushita et al., it was demonstrated that one in silico-predicted highly immunogenic neoantigen derived from a mutant spectrin-β2 is sufficient to induce tumor cell elimination in an unedited tumor.

Subsequent studies in a clinical setting have added further evidences for the ability of neoantigens to induce significant antitumoral immune responses and the predictability of such neoantigens by mutanome mining. Robbins and coworkers could identify neoantigens recognized by adoptively transferred tumor-reactive T cells mining exome sequencing data (Robbins et al. 2013), whereas van Rooji and colleagues discovered neoantigen-specific T cell reactivity in an ipilimumab-responsive melanoma by tumor exome analysis (van Rooij et al. 2013). Particularly, the correlation between successful immune checkpoint blockade and the occurrence of tumor-specific neoantigens has been demonstrated in several publications over the last years. Gubin and colleagues identified neoantigens following anti-PD1 or anti-CTLA-4 therapy of mice bearing progressively growing sarcoma. Additionally, they could show that therapeutic synthetic long-peptide vaccines incorporating these mutant epitopes are able to induce tumor rejection comparably to immune checkpoint blockade (Gubin et al. 2014). Even more interesting are the results of Snyder et al. and Rizvi et al. demonstrating a close correlation between the abundance of clonal neoantigens and sensitivity to immune checkpoint blockade by anti-PD1 or anti-CTLA-4 treatment in patients suffering from non-small-cell lung cancer or melanoma. Moreover, the predicted neoantigens elicited specific $CD8^+$ T cell responses in both studies (Snyder et al. 2014; Rizvi et al. 2015). Also for therapeutic approaches with adoptive tumor-infiltrating lymphocyte transfer in melanoma patients, a similar correlation between neoantigen load and therapy efficacy was revealed (Lu et al. 2014; Linnemann et al. 2015). Additionally, Tran and colleagues could provide evidence that immunotherapy based on mutation-specific $CD4^+$ T cells in a patient with epithelial cancer is possible (Tran et al. 2014).

The above-mentioned studies and several further publications demonstrated the feasibility of tumor exome mining plus immunogenicity prediction based on HLA allotypes and peptide-binding probability to identify patient-specific highly immunogenic neoantigens in different types of cancer with a variety of approaches (Rajasagi et al. 2014; Duan et al. 2014; Yadav et al. 2014; Tran et al. 2015). Moreover, the potential value of such neoantigens for personalized immunotherapy approaches has been frequently implied (Gubin et al. 2014; Tran et al. 2014). One possibility to target specifically neoantigens in cancer patients is to engineer neoantigen-specific T cell receptors and adoptively transfer these T cells (Leisegang et al. 2016) using methods also described here. A further option would be the immunization with vaccines incorporating the mutated sequences of neoantigens. The efficacy of such an immunization approach using peptides is currently under evaluation in a phase I clinical trial in IDH1R123H-mutated grade III–IV gliomas (NCT02454634). This clinical study is based on the results published by Schumacher and colleagues showing the antitumor potential of mutant IDH1 peptide vaccination in tumor-bearing MHC-humanized mice (Schumacher et al. 2014). However, mutant IDH1 seems to be a unique exception, since the mutation can be found frequently in diffuse grade II and grade III gliomas.

This high penetrance of a neoantigen appears to be in contrast to other tumor entities. In most human tumors, a large fraction of the mutations is not shared between patients at a meaningful frequency. Moreover, only a small portion of mutations within expressed genes have antigenic potential leading to T cell reactivity (Lu et al. 2014; Linnemann et al. 2015). Due to these limitations, broadly applicable neoantigens that can be used in huge patient cohorts for vaccinations are highly unlikely. Hence, mRNA vaccines represent a superior approach to satisfy the specific demands of a personalized immunotherapy based on neoantigens. The obvious advantages of mRNA vaccines in comparison with peptide vaccines were already mentioned above. Particularly, the production under well-defined and controlled conditions by in vitro transcription and the possibility to produce vaccines against different neoantigens by a common process and in a relatively short period of time fulfill the requirements for a personalized immunotherapy approach.

In a recent study of Kreiter and colleagues, the tumor-rejecting properties of neoantigen-based RNA vaccines were demonstrated in murine tumor models. In principle, mutanome analysis and MHC-binding prediction lead to selection of neoepitopes with proven in vivo immunogenicity for several of the selected neoepitopes. Additionally, the immunization of tumor-bearing mice with an mRNA vaccine coding for one B16-specific neoantigen resulted in a significantly increased survival of immunized mice in comparison with untreated mice. For the clinical setting, a combination of several neoantigens in one vaccine would be preferable to address tumor heterogeneity and immune editing which could mediate clinical failure of vaccines in humans. It was recently demonstrated that immunotherapy of CT26 lung metastasis after i.v. injection of tumor cells employing mRNA-encoded pentatope resulted in a drastic reduction of the tumor burden in the lung of vaccinated mice (Kreiter et al. 2015).

Based on these convincing results, a first phase I clinical trial was started in 2014 with melanoma patients, where a poly-neoepitope coding RNA vaccine is administered that targets the unique mutation signature of an individual patient (NCT02035956). In addition, a second clinical trial was set up in 2015 using a slightly different approach for the treatment of triple-negative breast cancer (NCT02316457).

In summary, induction of neoantigen-specific T cell reactivity via mRNA vaccines seems to be a promising strategy for successful cancer immunotherapies. Because of the tumor-restricted expression of the antigens that are being targeted, these personalized antitumor therapies offer the promise of high specificity and safety. Additionally, T cell reactivity that can be achieved with such personalized immunotherapies will further increase the spectrum of human malignancies that respond to cancer immunotherapy. Particularly, the correlation between immune checkpoint blockade and neoantigen burden implies synergistic effects by combination of personalized cancer immunotherapy with checkpoint blockade.

1.4 Cellular Vaccines: mRNA-Pulsed Dendritic Cells

mRNA-transfected dendritic cell (DC) vaccines represent a distinct type of vaccine strategy involving RNA. Among different types of antigen-presenting cells (APCs), DCs are considered to be the most potent ones because they can efficiently prime naïve T cells, thereby stimulating an adaptive immune response. Because of their ability to induce potent antitumor CTLs both in vitro and in vivo, DCs have been employed as cancer vaccination platform. The basis of this therapeutic strategy is to use cancer patient's DCs expressing tumor-associated antigens (TAAs) in order to activate antigen-specific T cells which after differentiation in cytotoxic effector T cells will be able to eradicate tumor cells, irrespective of their location. Moreover, these T cells can form an immunological memory providing in this way a defense against recurring cancer cells.

For the delivery of tumor antigens to DCs, mRNA is considered as an attractive vector as it overcomes some limitations associated with the use of antigen-derived peptides, the most commonly used strategy of antigen loading (Cerundolo et al. 2004; Schuler et al. 2003; Jager et al. 2002). Synthetic peptides represent only defined epitopes from known TAAs and are dependent on prior identification and on HLA restriction of the patients, meaning that the induced immune response by the vaccine is limited to the peptides used and that only patients with specific HLA allotypes can be treated (Van Nuffel et al. 2012). Instead, mRNA molecules can encode the entire tumor antigen. Therefore, multiple immunogenic epitopes within the same protein can be presented. In addition, since the protein is endogenously expressed and presented after mRNA transfection of DCs, multiple peptide–MHC complexes (pMHC) are generated; thereby, vaccine development is independent on the patient's genetic background.

Boczkowski and collaborators were the first ones to describe in the late 1990s that DCs pulsed with mRNA encoding for tumor antigens are potent antigen-presenting cells (Boczkowski et al. 1996). Only few years later, an early clinical trial using DCs loaded with RNA encoding the PSA proved the feasibility and safety of this approach. CTL responses against metastatic prostate tumors expressing PSA were indeed induced in some patients (Heiser et al. 2002). This approach was based on passive pulsing of DCs, which relies on the ability of these cells to take up mRNA through micropinocytosis (Diken et al. 2011). But this mechanism, involving transport into the endosomes, entails the risk that only a fraction of the mRNA can reach the cytosol and can then be translated into the protein. Therefore, several approaches have been established in order to deliver mRNA directly to the cytoplasm such as electroporation, nucleofection, lipofection, and more recently sonoporation (Benteyn et al. 2015). Above all, electroporation has been shown to be a powerful technique to introduce tumor antigens into DCs (Van Tendeloo et al. 2001).

mRNA encoding specific TAAs or total tumor RNA can be used to transfect DCs. Vaccine strategies employing DCs transfected with defined TAA mRNA avoid the need for growth of patient-specific tumor cells and reduce the risk of autoimmunity, which can be induced in patients by the presence of normally expressed self-proteins (Nair et al. 1999; Ponsaerts et al. 2003). However, there are some limitations due to the fact that for many cancers, the TAAs are unknown. An attractive alternative is to utilize DCs transfected with patient-derived total tumor RNA. Through this approach, the entire spectrum of tumor-specific antigens is displayed, thereby eliminating the need for identification of TAAs and allowing the immune system to use the most effective antigens while reducing the risk of escape mutants. Another advantage of using tumor-derived RNA as a source of whole-tumor antigen is that it can be quickly and easily amplified by RT-PCR from even a small amount of tumor (Heiser et al. 2002).

To date, several clinical trials have been reported using mRNA-transfected DCs. The majority of these studies have shown that tumor-specific T cell responses can be induced by mRNA-transfected DCs in several tumor entities such as brain cancer, melanoma, lung adenocarcinoma, renal cell carcinoma, and ovarian cancer (Bonehill et al. 2009; Caruso et al. 2004, 2005; Kyte et al. 2007; Nair et al. 2002; Su et al. 2003; Morse et al. 2003; Dannull et al. 2005; Van Nuffel et al. 2012). In particular, in the renal cell carcinoma study by Su et al., patients displayed no evidence of dose-limiting toxicity or induction of autoimmunity (Su et al. 2003).

Similarly, brain tumor and neuroblastoma studies conducted in nine and seven patients, respectively, showed a clinical response in a total of three of the patients.

Despite many progresses in mRNA-DC immunotherapies, clinical responses remain modest and new strategies on how to enhance the efficacy of mRNA-DC vaccines are being explored. Besides the delivery of tumor antigens, mRNA can be used to deliver also proteins that can modulate the function of DCs. Cotransfection of DCs with mRNA encoding TAAs and costimulatory molecules such as CD83 (Aerts-Toegaerr et al. 2007), OX40 (Dannull et al. 2005), and 4-1BBL (Grünebach et al. 2005) has shown to improve mRNA-DC vaccine efficacy in preclinical models. Moreover, DCs activated through electroporation with mRNAs encoding four tumor antigens as well as mRNAs encoding CD40 ligand and constitutively active TLR4 and CD70 (TriMix-DCs) resulted in a broad T cell response and durable tumor response in chemorefractory advanced melanoma patients (Van Nuffel et al. 2012). DCs have been also modified with mRNAs encoding immunomodulating cytokines. For example, DCs transfected with mRNAs encoding IL-12 and TAAs were shown to induce high-avidity cytotoxic T cells and enhance their effector function. In addition, the migratory capacity of DCs has been modulated using mRNA encoding a chimeric E/L-selectin, a strategy that led to increased migration of the DCs to lymph nodes upon intravenous administration (Dörrie et al. 2008).

Finally, further preclinical strategies have focused on increased DC function by coadministration of DCs transfected with TAA-encoding mRNAs or mRNAs encoding for antagonistic anti-CTLA-4 or agonistic anti-GITR antibodies (Pruitt et al. 2011). Thus, the engineered DCs have the ability not only to present the tumor antigen of interest but also to locally modulate immune checkpoints and the tumor microenvironment. Because of promising results in preclinical studies, this approach is currently under investigation in a phase I clinical trial for the treatment of melanoma patients (NCT01216436).

Taken together, these strategies have the potential to improve cancer immunotherapy.

1.5 CAR T Cells

Chimeric antigen receptor (CAR) T cell immunotherapy has recently emerged as a promising strategy for treating tumors (Cheadle et al. 2012; Restifo et al. 2012; Kershaw et al. 2013).

CAR T cells are a form of personalized cell therapy using patient-derived T cells. After the collection of T cells, they are genetically engineered to express receptors that allow them to recognize a specific antigen expressed by the patient's cancer cells and to attack the tumor, once the cells are infused back into the patient. Chimeric receptors are usually composed of an extracellular TAA-specific antibody-binding domain fused to intracellular T cell-signaling domains. CAR T cells can be engineered to target virtually any tumor-associated antigen (Jensen and Riddell 2015).

Since CARs are based on TAA-specific antibody-binding domains, recognition of the tumor antigen is HLA-independent, thereby extending its applicability to many patients and overcoming some tumor escape mechanisms (Ramos and Dotti 2011).

The adoptive transfer of genetically modified T cells engineered to express a CAR has shown early promising results in the treatment of hematologic malignancies (Kochenderfer et al. 2012; Brentjens et al. 2013; Porter et al. 2011; Grupp et al. 2013). However, by now, the use of CAR T cells was less successful for the therapy of solid cancers, one of the major issues being toxicity. Indeed, clinical trials have revealed the potential of engineered T cells to recognize and attack normal cells that share the expression of the tumor CAR-specific antigen, causing off-target toxicity (Lamers et al. 2006, 2013; Maus et al. 2013).

The main approach to modify the T cells uses viral vectors such as γ-retroviruses and lentiviruses that are expensive to produce and involve safety concerns associated with their integration into the genome (Kershaw et al. 2013).

Recently, mRNA electroporation has been used to engineer T cells with transient CAR expression. Prof. June and his colleagues at the University of Pennsylvania's Perelman School of Medicine were the first to prove the feasibility of this approach and the potential of mRNA-engineered T cells to induce robust antitumor effects in preclinical tumor models (Zhao et al. 2010; Barett et al. 2011, 2013).

Consequently, they conducted the first clinical trial to evaluate the feasibility and safety of repetitive infusions of mRNA CAR T cells in patients (Beatty et al. 2014). Two patients, one with advanced mesothelioma and the other one having metastatic pancreatic cancer, were recruited into a phase I clinical trial. Researchers used mRNA electroporation to engineer patient-derived T cells with a CAR specifically targeting mesothelin (Tmeso cells), a TAA overexpressed in several cancers. After ensuring their viability and specificity, engineered T cells were repetitively infused into the patients. Surprisingly, clinical and laboratory evidence of antitumor activity without explicit evidence of off-tumor toxicity against normal tissues was shown in both patients. In addition to the antitumor activity, CAR Tmeso cells were able to trigger a broad antitumor immune response consistent with epitope spreading. Moreover, mRNA CAR Tmeso cells were shown to persist transiently within the peripheral blood after intravenous administration and migrate to tumor tissue.

More recently, mRNA has been used not only to engineer T cells to recognize specific TAAs but also to transiently deliver a modified telomerase reverse transcriptase (TERT) to CD19 CAR T cells. This study provided an effective and safe method to extend the T cell replicative life span improving in this way the persistence and antitumor effects of CAR T cell in mouse xenograft tumor models of B cell malignancies compared with conventional CAR T cells (Bai et al. 2015).

All these findings support the development of mRNA-engineered T cells as a novel approach for adoptive cell transfer, providing a flexible platform for the treatment of cancer that may complement the use of retroviral and lentiviral engineered T cells.

2 Conclusion

The versatility of mRNA in encoding TAAs, patient-derived tumor neoantigens, or even chimeric antigen receptors makes mRNA vaccines a promising candidate for use in cancer immunotherapy. The encouraging results of the first clinical studies have prompted intensive research into strategies to increase the immunogenicity of the vaccines, which include modifications to the mRNA and the application or the combination with other treatments like checkpoint inhibitors or radiation therapy. These efforts will hopefully result in novel treatment options in cancer therapy, which will make full use of the unique properties of mRNA vaccines.

Acknowledgments We would like to thank Henoch Hong, Ulrike Gnad-Vogt, Ulrich Kruse, and Mariola Fotin-Mleczek for discussions and suggestions.

References

Aerts-Toegaert C, Heirman C, Tuyaerts S, Corthals J, Aerts JL, Bonehill A, Thielemans K, Breckpot K (2007) CD83 expression on dendritic cells and T cells: correlation with effective immune responses. Eur J Immunol 37(3):686–695

Anderson BR, Muramatsu H, Nallagatla SR, Bevilacqua PC, Sansing LH, Weissman D, Karikó K (2010) Incorporation of pseudouridine into mRNA enhances translation by diminishing PKR activation. Nucleic Acids Res 38(17):5884–5892

Bai Y, Kan S, Zhou S, Wang Y, Xu J, Cooke JP, Wen J, Deng H (2015) Enhancement of the in vivo persistence and antitumor efficacy of CD19 chimeric antigen receptor T cells through the delivery of modified TERT mRNA. Cell Discov 1:Article number: 15040

Barrett DM, Zhao Y, Liu X, Jiang S, Carpenito C, Kalos M, Carroll RG, June CH, Grupp SA (2011) Treatment of advanced leukemia in mice with mRNA engineered T cells. Hum Gene Ther 22(12):1575–1586

Barrett DM, Liu X, Jiang S, June CH, Grupp SA, Zhao Y (2013) Regimen-specific effects of RNA-modified chimeric antigen receptor T cells in mice with advanced leukemia. Hum Gene Ther 24(8):717–727

Beatty GL, Haas AR, Maus MV, Torigian DA, Soulen MC, Plesa G, Chew A, Zhao Y, Levine BL, Albelda SM, Kalos M, June CH (2014) Mesothelin-specific chimeric antigen receptor mRNA-engineered T cells induce anti-tumor activity in solid malignancies. Cancer Immunol Res 2(2):112–120

Benteyn D, Heirman C, Bonehill A, Thielemans K, Breckpot K (2015) mRNA-based dendritic cell vaccines. Expert Rev Vaccines 14(2):161–176

Boczkowski D, Nair SK, Snyder D, Gilboa E (1996) Dendritic cells pulsed with RNA are potent antigen-presenting cells in vitro and in vivo. J Exp Med 184(2):465–472

Bonehill A, Van Nuffel AM, Corthals J, Tuyaerts S, Heirman C, François V, Colau D, van der Bruggen P, Neyns B, Thielemans K (2009) Single-step antigen loading and activation of dendritic cells by mRNA electroporation for the purpose of therapeutic vaccination in melanoma patients. Clin Cancer Res 15(10):3366–3375

Boon T, Kellermann O (1977) Rejection by syngeneic mice of cell variants obtained by mutagenesis of a malignant teratocarcinoma cell line. Proc Natl Acad Sci USA 74(1):272–275

Boon T, Cerottini JC, Van den Eynde B, van der Bruggen P, Van Pel A (1994) Tumor antigens recognized by T lymphocytes. Annu Rev Immunol 12:337–365

Brentjens RJ, Davila ML, Riviere I, Park J, Wang X, Cowell LG, Bartido S, Stefanski J, Taylor C, Olszewska M, Borquez-Ojeda O, Qu J, Wasielewska T, He Q, Bernal Y, Rijo IV, Hedvat C, Kobos R, Curran K, Steinherz P, Jurcic J, Rosenblat T, Maslak P, Frattini M, Sadelain M (2013) CD19-targeted T cells rapidly induce molecular remissions in adults with chemotherapy-refractory acute lymphoblastic leukemia. Sci Transl Med 5(177):177ra38

Caruso DA, Orme LM, Neale AM, Radcliff FJ, Amor GM, Maixner W, Downie P, Hassall TE, Tang ML, Ashley DM (2004) Results of a phase 1 study utilizing monocyte-derived dendritic cells pulsed with tumor RNA in children and young adults with brain cancer. Neuro Oncol. 6 (3):236–246

Caruso DA, Orme LM, Amor GM, Neale AM, Radcliff FJ, Downie P, Tang ML, Ashley DM (2005) Results of a Phase I study utilizing monocyte-derived dendritic cells pulsed with tumor RNA in children with Stage 4 neuroblastoma. Cancer 103(6):1280–1291

Castle JC, Kreiter S, Diekmann J, Löwer M, van de Roemer N, de Graaf J, Selmi A, Diken M, Boegel S, Paret C, Koslowski M, Kuhn AN, Britten CM, Huber C, Türeci O, Sahin U (2012) Exploiting the mutanome for tumor vaccination. Cancer Res 72(5):1081–1091

Cerundolo V, Hermans IF, Salio M (2004) Dendritic cells: a journey from laboratory to clinic. Nat Immunol 5(1):7–10

Cheadle EJ, Sheard V, Hombach AA, Chmielewski M, Riet T, Berrevoets C, Schooten E, Lamers C, Abken H, Debets R, Gilham DE (2012) Chimeric antigen receptors for T-cell based therapy. Methods Mol Biol 907:645–666

Coulie PG, Lehmann F, Lethé B, Herman J, Lurquin C, Andrawiss M, Boon T (1995) A mutated intron sequence codes for an antigenic peptide recognized by cytolytic T lymphocytes on a human melanoma. Proc Natl Acad Sci U S A. 92(17):7976–7980

Dannull J, Nair S, Su Z, Boczkowski D, DeBeck C, Yang B, Gilboa E, Vieweg J (2005) Enhancing the immunostimulatory function of dendritic cells by transfection with mRNA encoding OX40 ligand. Blood 105(8):3206–3213

Demaria S, Formenti SC (2012) Role of T lymphocytes in tumor response to radiotherapy. Front Oncol 2:95

Diken M, Kreiter S, Selmi A, Britten CM, Huber C, Türeci Ö, Sahin U (2011) Selective uptake of naked vaccine RNA by dendritic cells is driven by macropinocytosis and abrogated upon DC maturation. Gene Ther 18(7):702–708

Dörrie J, Schaft N, Müller I, Wellner V, Schunder T, Hänig J, Oostingh GJ, Schön MP, Robert C, Kämpgen E, Schuler G (2008) Introduction of functional chimeric E/L-selectin by RNA electroporation to target dendritic cells from blood to lymph nodes. Cancer Immunol Immunother 57(4):467–477

Duan F, Duitama J, Al Seesi S, Ayres CM, Corcelli SA, Pawashe AP, Blanchard T, McMahon D, Sidney J, Sette A, Baker BM, Mandoiu II, Srivastava PK (2014) Genomic and bioinformatic profiling of mutational neoepitopes reveals new rules to predict anticancer immunogenicity. J Exp Med 211(11):2231–2248

Echchakir H, Mami-Chouaib F, Vergnon I, Baurain JF, Karanikas V, Chouaib S, Coulie PG (2001) A point mutation in the alpha-actinin-4 gene generates an antigenic peptide recognized by autologous cytolytic T lymphocytes on a human lung carcinoma. Cancer Res 61(10):4078–4083

Formenti SC, Demaria S (2013) Combining radiotherapy and cancer immunotherapy: a paradigm shift. J Natl Cancer Inst 105(4):256–265

Fotin-Mleczek M, Duchardt KM, Lorenz C, Pfeiffer R, Ojkić-Zrna S, Probst J, Kallen KJ (2011) Messenger RNA-based vaccines with dual activity induce balanced TLR-7 dependent adaptive immune responses and provide antitumor activity. J Immunother 34(1):1–15

Fotin-Mleczek M, Zanzinger K, Heidenreich R, Lorenz C, Thess A, Duchardt KM, Kallen KJ (2012) Highly potent mRNA based cancer vaccines represent an attractive platform for combination therapies supporting an improved therapeutic effect. J Gene Med. 14(6):428–439

Fotin-Mleczek M, Zanzinger K, Heidenreich R, Lorenz C, Kowalczyk A, Kallen KJ, Huber SM (2014) mRNA-based vaccines synergize with radiation therapy to eradicate established tumors. Radiat Oncol 9:180

Garnett CT, Schlom J, Hodge JW (2008) Combination of docetaxel and recombinant vaccine enhances T-cell responses and antitumor activity: effects of docetaxel on immune enhancement. Clin Cancer Res 14(11):3536–3544

Gerlinger M, Catto JW, Orntoft TF, Real FX, Zwarthoff EC, Swanton C (2015) Intratumour heterogeneity in urologic cancers: from molecular evidence to clinical implications. Eur Urol 67(4):729–737

Golden EB, Frances D, Pellicciotta I, Demaria S, Helen Barcellos-Hoff M, Formenti SC (2014) Radiation fosters dose-dependent and chemotherapy-induced immunogenic cell death. Oncoimmunology 3:e28518

Grünebach F, Kayser K, Weck MM, Müller MR, Appel S, Brossart P (2005) Cotransfection of dendritic cells with RNA coding for HER-2/neu and 4-1BBL increases the induction of tumor antigen specific cytotoxic T lymphocytes. Cancer Gene Ther 12(9):749–756

Grupp SA, Kalos M, Barrett D, Aplenc R, Porter DL, Rheingold SR, Teachey DT, Chew A, Hauck B, Wright JF, Milone MC, Levine BL, June CH (2013) Chimeric antigen receptor-modified T cells for acute lymphoid leukemia. N Engl J Med 368(16):1509–1518

Gubin MM, Zhang X, Schuster H, Caron E, Ward JP, Noguchi T, Ivanova Y, Hundal J, Arthur CD, Krebber WJ, Mulder GE, Toebes M, Vesely MD, Lam SS, Korman AJ, Allison JP, Freeman GJ, Sharpe AH, Pearce EL, Schumacher TN, Aebersold R, Rammensee HG, Melief CJ, Mardis ER, Gillanders WE, Artyomov MN, Schreiber RD (2014) Checkpoint blockade cancer immunotherapy targets tumour-specific mutant antigens. Nature 515 (7528):577–581

Heiser A, Coleman D, Dannull J, Yancey D, Maurice MA, Lallas CD, Dahm P, Niedzwiecki D, Gilboa E, Vieweg J (2002) Autologous dendritic cells transfected with prostate-specific antigen RNA stimulate CTL responses against metastatic prostate tumors. J Clin Invest. 109 (3):409–417

Hoerr I, Obst R, Rammensee HG, Jung G (2000) In vivo application of RNA leads to induction of specific cytotoxic T lymphocytes and antibodies. Eur J Immunol 30(1):1–7

Jäger E, Jäger D, Knuth A (2002) Clinical cancer vaccine trials. Curr Opin Immunol 14 (2):178–182

Jensen MC, Riddell SR (2015) Designing chimeric antigen receptors to effectively and safely target tumors. Curr Opin Immunol 33:9–15

Kallen KJ, Theß A (2014) A development that may evolve into a revolution in medicine: mRNA as the basis for novel, nucleotide-based vaccines and drugs. Ther Adv Vaccines. 2(1):10–31

Kallen KJ, Heidenreich R, Schnee M, Petsch B, Schlake T, Thess A, Baumhof P, Scheel B, Koch SD, Fotin-Mleczek M (2013) A novel, disruptive vaccination technology: self-adjuvanted RNActive(®) vaccines. Hum Vaccin Immunother. 9(10):2263–2276

Kantoff PW, Higano CS, Shore ND, Berger ER, Small EJ, Penson DF, Redfern CH, Ferrari AC, Dreicer R, Sims RB, Xu Y, Frohlich MW, Schellhammer PF; IMPACT Study Investigators (2010) Sipuleucel-T immunotherapy for castration-resistant prostate cancer. N Engl J Med. 363 (5):411–22

Karikó K, Muramatsu H, Welsh FA, Ludwig J, Kato H, Akira S, Weissman D (2008) Incorporation of pseudouridine into mRNA yields superior nonimmunogenic vector with increased translational capacity and biological stability. Mol Ther 16(11):1833–1840

Kershaw MH, Westwood JA, Darcy PK (2013) Gene-engineered T cells for cancer therapy. Nat Rev Cancer 13(8):525–541

Knapp DC, Mata JE, Reddy MT, Devi GR, Iversen PL (2003) Resistance to chemotherapeutic drugs overcome by c-Myc inhibition in a Lewis lung carcinoma murine model. Anticancer Drugs 14:39–47

Kochenderfer JN, Dudley ME, Feldman SA, Wilson WH, Spaner DE, Maric I, Stetler-Stevenson M, Phan GQ, Hughes MS, Sherry RM, Yang JC, Kammula US, Devillier L, Carpenter R, Nathan DA, Morgan RA, Laurencot C, Rosenberg SA (2012) B-cell depletion and remissions of malignancy along with cytokine-associated toxicity in a clinical trial of anti-CD19 chimeric-antigen-receptor-transduced T cells. Blood 119(12):2709–2720

Kowalczyk A, Doener F, Zanzinger K, Noth J, Baumhof P, Fotin-Mleczek M, Heidenreich R (2016) Self-adjuvanted mRNA vaccines induce local innate immune responses that lead to a potent and boostable adaptive immunity. Vaccine 34:3882–3893

Kreiter S, Vormehr M, van de Roemer N, Diken M, Löwer M, Diekmann J, Boegel S, Schrörs B, Vascotto F, Castle JC, Tadmor AD, Schoenberger SP, Huber C, Türeci Ö, Sahin U (2015) Mutant MHC class II epitopes drive therapeutic immune responses to cancer. Nature 520 (7549):692–696

Kübler H, Scheel B, Gnad-Vogt U, Miller K, Schultze-Seemann W, Vom Dorp F, Parmiani G, Hampel C, Wedel S, Trojan L, Jocham D, Maurer T, Rippin G, Fotin-Mleczek M, von der Mülbe F, Probst J, Hoerr I, Kallen KJ, Lander T, Stenzl A (2015) Self-adjuvanted mRNA vaccination in advanced prostate cancer patients: a first-in-man phase I/IIa study. J Immunother Cancer 3:26

Kyte JA, Kvalheim G, Lislerud K, thor Straten P, Dueland S, Aamdal S, Gaudernack G (2007) T cell responses in melanoma patients after vaccination with tumor-mRNA transfected dendritic cells. Cancer Immunol Immunother 56(5):659–675

Lamers CH, Sleijfer S, Vulto AG, Kruit WH, Kliffen M, Debets R, Gratama JW, Stoter G, Oosterwijk E (2006) Treatment of metastatic renal cell carcinoma with autologous T-lymphocytes genetically retargeted against carbonic anhydrase IX: first clinical experience. J Clin Oncol 24(13):e20–e22

Lamers CH, Sleijfer S, van Steenbergen S, van Elzakker P, van Krimpen B, Groot C, Vulto A, den Bakker M, Oosterwijk E, Debets R, Gratama JW (2013) Treatment of metastatic renal cell carcinoma with CAIX CAR-engineered T cells: clinical evaluation and management of on-target toxicity. Mol Ther 21(4):904–912

Leisegang M, Kammertoens T, Uckert W, Blankenstein T (2016) Targeting human melanoma neoantigens by T cell receptor gene therapy. J Clin Invest 126(3):854–858

Linnemann C, van Buuren MM, Bies L, Verdegaal EM, Schotte R, Calis JJ, Behjati S, Velds A, Hilkmann H, Atmioui DE, Visser M, Stratton MR, Haanen JB, Spits H, van der Burg SH, Schumacher TN (2015) High-throughput epitope discovery reveals frequent recognition of neo-antigens by CD4+ T cells in human melanoma. Nat Med 21(1):81–85

Lu YC, Yao X, Crystal JS, Li YF, El-Gamil M, Gross C, Davis L, Dudley ME, Yang JC, Samuels Y, Rosenberg SA, Robbins PF (2014) Efficient identification of mutated cancer antigens recognized by T cells associated with durable tumor regressions. Clin Cancer Res 20 (13):3401–3410

Lurquin C, Van Pel A, Mariamé B, De Plaen E, Szikora JP, Janssens C, Reddehase MJ, Lejeune J, Boon T (1989) Structure of the gene of tum- transplantation antigen P91A: the mutated exon encodes a peptide recognized with Ld by cytolytic T cells. Cell 58(2):293–303

Mandelboim O, Vadai E, Fridkin M, Katz-Hillel A, Feldman M, Berke G, Eisenbach L (1995) Regression of established murine carcinoma metastases following vaccination with tumour-associated antigen peptides. Nat Med 1(11):1179–1183

Martincorena I, Roshan A, Gerstung M, Ellis P, Van Loo P, McLaren S, Wedge DC, Fullam A, Alexandrov LB, Tubio JM, Stebbings L, Menzies A, Widaa S, Stratton MR, Jones PH, Campbell PJ (2015) High burden and pervasive positive selection of somatic mutations in normal human skin. Science 348(6237):880–886 Tumor evolution

Martinon F, Krishnan S, Lenzen G, Magné R, Gomard E, Guillet JG, Lévy JP, Meulien P (1993) Induction of virus-specific cytotoxic T lymphocytes in vivo by liposome-entrapped mRNA. Eur J Immunol 23(7):1719–1722

Matsushita H, Vesely MD, Koboldt DC, Rickert CG, Uppaluri R, Magrini VJ, Arthur CD, White JM, Chen YS, Shea LK, Hundal J, Wendl MC, Demeter R, Wylie T, Allison JP, Smyth MJ, Old LJ, Mardis ER, Schreiber RD (2012) Cancer exome analysis reveals a T-cell-dependent mechanism of cancer immunoediting. Nature 482(7385):400–404

Maus MV, Haas AR, Beatty GL, Albelda SM, Levine BL, Liu X, Zhao Y, Kalos M, June CH (2013) T cells expressing chimeric antigen receptors can cause anaphylaxis in humans. Cancer Immunol Res 1(1):26–31

Melero I, Berman DM, Aznar MA, Korman AJ, Pérez Gracia JL, Haanen J (2015) Evolving synergistic combinations of targeted immunotherapies to combat cancer. Nat Rev Cancer 15 (8):457–472
Moore MW, Carbone FR, Bevan MJ (1988) Introduction of soluble protein into the class I pathway of antigen processing and presentation. Cell 54(6):777–785
Morse MA, Nair SK, Mosca PJ, Hobeika AC, Clay TM, Deng Y, Boczkowski D, Proia A, Neidzwiecki D, Clavien PA, Hurwitz HI, Schlom J, Gilboa E, Lyerly HK (2003) Immunotherapy with autologous, human dendritic cells transfected with carcinoembryonic antigen mRNA. Cancer Invest 21(3):341–349
Nair SK, Hull S, Coleman D, Gilboa E, Lyerly HK, Morse MA (1999) Induction of carcinoembryonic antigen (CEA)-specific cytotoxic T-lymphocyte responses in vitro using autologous dendritic cells loaded with CEA peptide or CEA RNA in patients with metastatic malignancies expressing CEA. Int J Cancer 82(1):121–124
Nair SK, Morse M, Boczkowski D, Cumming RI, Vasovic L, Gilboa E, Lyerly HK (2002) Induction of tumor-specific cytotoxic T lymphocytes in cancer patients by autologous tumor RNA-transfected dendritic cells. Ann Surg 235(4):540–549
Palmer M, Parker J, Modi S, Butts C, Smylie M, Meikle A, Kehoe M, MacLean G, Longenecker M (2001) Phase I study of the BLP25 (MUC1 peptide) liposomal vaccine for active specific immunotherapy in stage IIIB/IV non-small-cell lung cancer. Clin Lung Cancer 3 (1):49–57 discussion 58
Petsch B, Schnee M, Vogel AB, Lange E, Hoffmann B, Voss D, Schlake T, Thess A, Kallen KJ, Stitz L, Kramps T (2012) Protective efficacy of in vitro synthesized, specific mRNA vaccines against influenza A virus infection. Nat Biotechnol 30(12):1210–1216
Ponsaerts P, Van Tendeloo VF, Berneman ZN (2003) Cancer immunotherapy using RNA-loaded dendritic cells. Clin Exp Immunol 134(3):378–384
Porter DL, Levine BL, Kalos M, Bagg A, June CH (2011) Chimeric antigen receptor-modified T cells in chronic lymphoid leukemia. N Engl J Med 365(8):725–733
Pruitt SK, Boczkowski D, de Rosa N, Haley NR, Morse MA, Tyler DS, Dannull J, Nair S (2011) Enhancement of anti-tumor immunity through local modulation of CTLA-4 and GITR by dendritic cells. Eur J Immunol 41(12):3553–3563
Rajasagi M, Shukla SA, Fritsch EF, Keskin DB, DeLuca D, Carmona E, Zhang W, Sougnez C, Cibulskis K, Sidney J, Stevenson K, Ritz J, Neuberg D, Brusic V, Gabriel S, Lander ES, Getz G, Hacohen N, Wu CJ (2014) Systematic identification of personal tumor-specific neoantigens in chronic lymphocytic leukemia. Blood 124(3):453–462
Rammensee HG (2006) Some considerations on the use of peptides and mRNA for therapeutic vaccination against cancer. Immunol Cell Biol 84(3):290–294
Ramos CA, Dotti G (2011) Chimeric antigen receptor (CAR)-engineered lymphocytes for cancer therapy. Expert Opin Biol Ther 11(7):855–873
Reits EA, Hodge JW, Herberts CA, Groothuis TA, Chakraborty M, Wansley EK, Camphausen K, Luiten RM, de Ru AH, Neijssen J, Griekspoor A, Mesman E, Verreck FA, Spits H, Schlom J, van Veelen P, Neefjes JJ (2006) Radiation modulates the peptide repertoire, enhances MHC class I expression, and induces successful antitumor immunotherapy. J Exp Med 203(5):1259–1271
Restifo NP, Dudley ME, Rosenberg SA (2012) Adoptive immunotherapy for cancer: harnessing the T cell response. Nat Rev Immunol 12(4):269–281
Rizvi NA, Hellmann MD, Snyder A, Kvistborg P, Makarov V, Havel JJ, Lee W, Yuan J, Wong P, Ho TS, Miller ML, Rekhtman N, Moreira AL, Ibrahim F, Bruggeman C, Gasmi B, Zappasodi R, Maeda Y, Sander C, Garon EB, Merghoub T, Wolchok JD, Schumacher TN, Chan TA (2015) Cancer immunology. Mutational landscape determines sensitivity to PD-1 blockade in non-small cell lung cancer. Science 348(6230):124–128
Robbins PF, Lu YC, El-Gamil M, Li YF, Gross C, Gartner J, Lin JC, Teer JK, Cliften P, Tycksen E, Samuels Y, Rosenberg SA (2013) Mining exomic sequencing data to identify mutated antigens recognized by adoptively transferred tumor-reactive T cells. Nat Med 19 (6):747–752

Savai R, Schermuly RT, Pullamsetti SS, Schneider M, Greschus S, Ghofrani HA, Traupe H, Grimminger F, Banat GA (2007) A combination hybrid-based vaccination/adoptive cellular therapy to prevent tumor growth by involvement of T cells. Cancer Res 67(11):5443–5453
Scheel B, Teufel R, Probst J, Carralot JP, Geginat J, Radsak M, Jarrossay D, Wagner H, Jung G, Rammensee HG, Hoerr I, Pascolo S (2005) Toll-like receptor-dependent activation of several human blood cell types by protamine-condensed mRNA. Eur J Immunol 35(5):1557–1566
Schnee M, Vogel AB, Voss D, Petsch B, Baumhof P, Kramps T, Stitz L (2016) An mRNA vaccine encoding rabies virus glycoprotein induces protection against lethal infection in mice and correlates of protection in adult and newborn Pigs. PLoS Negl Trop Dis 10(6)
Schuler G, Schuler-Thurner B, Steinman RM (2003) The use of dendritic cells in cancer immunotherapy. Curr Opin Immunol 15(2):138–147
Schumacher TN, Schreiber RD (2015) Neoantigens in cancer immunotherapy. Science 348 (6230):69–74
Schumacher T, Bunse L, Pusch S, Sahm F, Wiestler B, Quandt J, Menn O, Osswald M, Oezen I, Ott M, Keil M, Balß J, Rauschenbach K, Grabowska AK, Vogler I, Diekmann J, Trautwein N, Eichmüller SB, Okun J, Stevanović S, Riemer AB, Sahin U, Friese MA, Beckhove P, von Deimling A, Wick W, Platten M (2014) A vaccine targeting mutant IDH1 induces antitumour immunity. Nature 512(7514):324–327
Sebastian M, Papachristofilou A, Weiss C, Früh M, Cathomas R, Hilbe W, Wehler T, Rippin G, Koch SD, Scheel B, Fotin-Mleczek M, Heidenreich R, Kallen KJ, Gnad-Vogt U, Zippelius A (2014) Phase Ib study evaluating a self-adjuvanted mRNA cancer vaccine (RNActive®) combined with local radiation as consolidation and maintenance treatment for patients with stage IV non-small cell lung cancer. BMC Cancer 14:748
Shojaei F, Wu X, Malik AK, Zhong C, Baldwin ME, Schanz S, Fuh G, Gerber H-P, Ferrara N (2007) Tumor refractoriness to anti-VEGF treatment is mediated by CD11b+ Gr1+ myeloid cells. Nat Biotechnol 25:911–920
Snyder A, Makarov V, Merghoub T, Yuan J, Zaretsky JM, Desrichard A, Walsh LA, Postow MA, Wong P, Ho TS, Hollmann TJ, Bruggeman C, Kannan K, Li Y, Elipenahli C, Liu C, Harbison CT, Wang L, Ribas A, Wolchok JD, Chan TA (2014) Genetic basis for clinical response to CTLA-4 blockade in melanoma. N Engl J Med 371(23):2189–2199
Stratton MR (2011) Exploring the genomes of cancer cells: progress and promise. Science 331 (6024):1553–1558
Su Z, Dannull J, Heiser A, Yancey D, Pruitt S, Madden J, Coleman D, Niedzwiecki D, Gilboa E, Vieweg J (2003) Immunological and clinical responses in metastatic renal cancer patients vaccinated with tumor RNA-transfected dendritic cells. Cancer Res 63(9):2127–2133
Tran E, Turcotte S, Gros A, Robbins PF, Lu YC, Dudley ME, Wunderlich JR, Somerville RP, Hogan K, Hinrichs CS, Parkhurst MR, Yang JC, Rosenberg SA (2014) Cancer immunotherapy based on mutation-specific CD4+ T cells in a patient with epithelial cancer. Science 344 (6184):641–645
Tran E, Ahmadzadeh M, Lu YC, Gros A, Turcotte S, Robbins PF, Gartner JJ, Zheng Z, Li YF, Ray S, Wunderlich JR, Somerville RP, Rosenberg SA (2015) Immunogenicity of somatic mutations in human gastrointestinal cancers. Science 350(6266):1387–1390
Van den Eynde B, Lethé B, Van Pel A, De Plaen E, Boon T (1991) The gene coding for a major tumor rejection antigen of tumor P815 is identical to the normal gene of syngeneic DBA/2 mice. J Exp Med 173(6):1373–1384
van der Bruggen P, Traversari C, Chomez P, Lurquin C, De Plaen E, Van den Eynde B, Knuth A, Boon T (1991) A gene encoding an antigen recognized by cytolytic T lymphocytes on a human melanoma. Science 254(5038):1643–1647
Van Nuffel AM, Wilgenhof S, Thielemans K, Bonehill A (2012) Overcoming HLA restriction in clinical trials: Immune monitoring of mRNA-loaded DC therapy. Oncoimmunology 1 (8):1392–1394
van Rooij N, van Buuren MM, Philips D, Velds A, Toebes M, Heemskerk B, van Dijk LJ, Behjati S, Hilkmann H, El Atmioui D, Nieuwland M, Stratton MR, Kerkhoven RM, Kesmir C,

Haanen JB, Kvistborg P, Schumacher TN (2013) Tumor exome analysis reveals neoantigen-specific T-cell reactivity in an ipilimumab-responsive melanoma. J Clin Oncol 31(32):e439–e442

Van Tendeloo VF, Ponsaerts P, Lardon F, Nijs G, Lenjou M, Van Broeckhoven C, Van Bockstaele DR, Berneman ZN (2001) Highly efficient gene delivery by mRNA electroporation in human hematopoietic cells: superiority to lipofection and passive pulsing of mRNA and to electroporation of plasmid cDNA for tumor antigen loading of dendritic cells. Blood 98 (1):49–56

Vesely MD, Schreiber RD (2013) Cancer immunoediting: antigens, mechanisms, and implications to cancer immunotherapy. Ann NY Acad Sci 1284:1–5

Wölfel T, Hauer M, Schneider J, Serrano M, Wölfel C, Klehmann-Hieb E, De Plaen E, Hankeln T, Meyer zum Büschenfelde KH, Beach D (1995) A p16INK4a-insensitive CDK4 mutant targeted by cytolytic T lymphocytes in a human melanoma. Science 269(5228):1281–1284

Wolff JA, Malone RW, Williams P, Chong W, Acsadi G, Jani A, Felgner PL (1990) Direct gene transfer into mouse muscle in vivo. Science 247(4949 Pt 1):1465–1468

Yadav M, Jhunjhunwala S, Phung QT, Lupardus P, Tanguay J, Bumbaca S, Franci C, Cheung TK, Fritsche J, Weinschenk T, Modrusan Z, Mellman I, Lill JR, Delamarre L (2014) Predicting immunogenic tumour mutations by combining mass spectrometry and exome sequencing. Nature 515(7528):572–576

Zhao Y, Moon E, Carpenito C, Paulos CM, Liu X, Brennan AL, Chew A, Carroll RG, Scholler J, Levine BL, Albelda SM, June CH (2010) Multiple injections of electroporated autologous T cells expressing a chimeric antigen receptor mediate regression of human disseminated tumor. Cancer Res 70(22):9053–9061

Gene Therapeutic Approaches to Overcome ABCB1-Mediated Drug Resistance

Hermann Lage

Abstract

Multidrug resistance (MDR) to pharmaceutical active agents is a common clinical problem in patients suffering from cancer. MDR is often mediated by over expression of trans-membrane xenobiotic transport molecules belonging to the superfamily of ATP-binding cassette (ABC)-transporters. This protein family includes the classical MDR-associated transporter ABCB1 (MDR1/P-gp). Inhibition of ABC-transporters by low molecular weight compounds in cancer patients has been extensively investigated in clinical trials, but the results have been disappointing. Thus, in the last decades alternative experimental therapeutic strategies for overcoming MDR were under extensive investigation. These include gene therapeutic approaches applying antisense-, ribozyme-, RNA interference-, and CRISPR/Cas9-based techniques. Various delivery strategies were used to reverse MDR in different tumor models in vitro and in vivo. Results and conclusions of these gene therapeutic studies will be discussed.

Keywords

Multidrug resistance · Cancer · Gene therapy · RNA interference · CRISPR/Cas9

H. Lage (✉)
Fachbereich Pathologie, Vivantes Klinikum Neukölln, Rudower Allee 48, 12351 Berlin, Germany
e-mail: hermann.lage@vivantes.de

W. Walther (ed.), *Current Strategies in Cancer Gene Therapy*,
Recent Results in Cancer Research 209, DOI 10.1007/978-3-319-42934-2_6

1 Introduction

Resistance including multidrug resistance (MDR) to chemotherapy is a common clinical problem in patients suffering from cancer. Besides alterations in various cellular pathways involved in regulation of cell cycle, apoptosis, and repair, MDR is often mediated by over expression of trans-membrane xenobiotic transport molecules belonging to the superfamily of ATP-binding cassette (ABC)-transporters (Lage 2008). The first identified member of this family involved in MDR was ABCB1, a 170 kDa cytoplasm membrane-embedded glycoprotein also known as P-glycoprotein, P170, or MDR1/P-gp (Juliano and Ling 1976). Following the identification of ABCB1, a large number of drug-extruding ABC-transporters have been identified in cancer cells. Inhibition of ABC-transporters by low molecular weight compounds in cancer patients has been extensively investigated in clinical trials, but the results have been disappointing. In particular, different experimental therapeutic strategies were developed which are able to selectively switch off specific ABC-transporter encoding genes in drug-resistant cancer cells. The most promising of these efforts focussed on the design of RNA-based therapeutics.

Already in the 1980s, DNA- and RNA-based antisense oligonucleotides with different chemical modifications were tested with different model systems both in vitro and in vivo with varying degrees of success. Accordingly, at that time the synthesis of ABCB1 could be inhibited by nonionic oligonucleoside methylphosphonates in human multidrug-resistant K562 erythroleukemia cells (Vasanthakumar and Ahmed 1989).

During the 1990s, ribozymes with both antisense and catalytic properties were successfully applied for specific knock down of gene expression. Ribozymes were demonstrated to selectively inhibit the expression of various genes including the ABCB1 encoding gene in human cancer cell lines (Kobayashi et al. 1994; Holm et al. 1994) as well as in tumors grown in mice (Gao et al. 1999). However, unsolved problems with delivery issues for these therapeutic RNA molecules limited their clinical exploitation.

In the 2000s, advances have revealed new opportunities for the development of RNA therapeutics in particular those based on the utilization of the RNA interference (RNAi) pathway. The observation that synthetic RNA molecules, i.e., double-stranded small interfering RNA (siRNA) molecules, could be used to specifically silence genes in mammalian cells (Elbashir et al. 2001) initiated an explosion of research on the mechanisms and application of the RNAi phenomenon. Following the first evidence of the in vivo efficacy of the RNAi technology in an animal model (Soutschek et al. 2004), RNA-based drugs were developed efforts and several clinical trials, including phase III trials, started with RNAi-based therapeutics (Whitehead et al. 2009). Following the first proofs that this technology is useful to circumvent MDR by inhibition of ABCB1 synthesis (Nieth et al. 2003; Wu et al. 2003), a huge number of studies were published applying this technique in different cancer cell models in vitro and in vivo.

At the beginning of the 2010s, the development of the CRISPR/Cas9-gene editing technology offered new possibilities as a general tool for the precise regulation of gene expression in eukaryotic cells (Gilbert et al. 2013). In cancer research, firstly this technique was applied in vitro to target and destroy the HPV16-encoded E6 or E7 genes in human cervical carcinoma cells resulting in cell cycle arrest leading to cancer cell death (Kennedy et al. 2014). So far, only a single study was published in which this new technology was applied to silence ABCB1 expression in a canine in vitro model (Simoff et al. 2016). In this study, Madin–Darby canine kidney cells (MDCK II wt) showing high expression of ABCB1 were transfected with CRISPR/Cas9 plasmid vectors, targeting three specific regions of the ABCB1 encoding gene. The treated cells completely lacked detectable levels of ABCB1 expression and no ABCB1-specific transport activity could be observed.

Just like with antisense oligonucleotides and ribozymes, the key challenge with RNAi-based or CRISPR/Cas9-based therapeutics is achieving the effective delivery. Naked RNA molecules are rapidly degraded in physiological milieu and, therefore, have very short half-life times. Former chemical modifications which were developed to prolong the half-life of antisense molecules and ribozymes have proved to be valuable in developing siRNA therapeutics. Most of these modifications concerned to the oligonucleotide backbone linkages to protect against degradation by nucleases. RNAi or CRISPR/Cas9 strategies may offer greater opportunities than those resulting from earlier approaches, potentially as a consequence of the possibility by which the hurdle of delivery will be solved. However, new approaches for delivery of therapeutic RNA molecules are continuously in development and were applied for targeting MDR-associated ABC-transporters.

2 Resistance Overcoming Gene Therapy Approaches

2.1 Delivery by Transfection

The easiest way for the delivery of therapeutic agents consisting of nucleic acids is transfection using different types of transfection reagents. These reagents consist of cationic lipids or other cationic polymers which can form complexes with negatively charged nucleic acids. These complexes are admitted by the target cells via endocytosis. Respectively to the complex-forming reagent this process is designated as lipofection or polyfection. Accordingly, the first studies using antisense oligonucleotides, ribozymes, or RNAi-mediating agents applied transfection procedures for knock down of the ABCB1-encoding mRNA. Meanwhile, a huge number of studies using different cell models were published (overview in Lage 2009). Depending on the cell models, the gene silencing agents, and the target sequences, a wide range of efficacies in gene silencing could be observed. As an example, treatment of the multidrug-resistant human gastric carcinoma cell line EPG85-257RDB and the human pancreatic carcinoma cell line EPP85-181RDB with complexes consisting of chemically synthesized siRNAs and cationic polymers resulted in up to 90 % decrease in the ABCB1 mRNA expression level (Nieth et al. 2003). In this transient experiment, resistance against the ABCB1 substrate daunorubicin was decreased to 89 % (EPP85-181RDB) or 58 % (EPG85-257RDB). However, experiments with these cell models applying stable transfection procedures showed more efficacies in reversal of MDR. ABCB1 downregulation by transfection with anti-ABCB1 ribozyme or anti-ABCB1 short hairpin RNA (shRNA)-plasmid-based expression vectors resulted in each case in a comprehensive knock down of the ABCB1 mRNA expression and a complete reversal of the multidrug-resistant phenotype in EPP85-181RDB and EPG85-257RDB cells (Stege et al. 2004).

Different improvements of these strategies were developed. For example a "multitarget multiribozyme" (MTMR) was constructed (Kowalski et al. 2005). This MTMR was simultaneous directed against the mRNAs encoding three different ABC-transporters, i.e., against ABCB1, ABCC2, and ABCG2. In this MTMR, the three trans-acting hammerhead ribozymes directed against ABCB1, ABCC2, and ABCG2 were linked with ABCB1-homologous spacer sequences and three cis-acting ABCB1-specific ribozymes. The trans-acting hammerhead ribozymes were liberated from the MTMR through autocatalytic self-cleavage by the cis-acting ribozymes. In different cell models, the MTMR could cleave their specific substrates without loss of efficiency when compared with the corresponding monoribozymes.

Although these studies demonstrated the high potential of gene therapeutic approaches for reversal of MDR by targeting ABCB1, these experimental strategies are not suitable for therapeutic application. Thus, improved delivery protocols were developed.

2.2 Nanoparticle-Based Delivery

Different types of nanocarriers designed for gene therapy including RNA-based drugs therapy have been developed (Xu et al. 2014). These carriers include liposomes, metallic and polymeric nanoparticles, dendrimers, gelatins, and quantum dots/rods each showing distinct characteristics. Modulation of classical ABCB1-mediated MDR by nanoparticle-based siRNA delivery started in 2005 with construction of a delivery vehicle consisting of a dendrimer conjugated to Tat peptide, a cell penetrating peptide (Kang et al. 2005). However, the dendrimer–oligonucleotide complexes were poorly effective for delivery of siRNAs and expression of ABCB1 was only inhibited weakly. In the next nanoparticle-based RNAi approaches, an improvement of the efficacy of ABCB1 inhibition could be observed (Patil et al. 2010; Susa et al. 2010). Several studies followed using different multidrug-resistant cancer cell models for in vitro and in vivo studies (Yin et al. 2012; Zhao et al. 2013; Nourbakhsh et al. 2015; Yang et al. 2015). All these studies provide a proof of concept that this technique may be applicable for circumvention of ABCB1-associated MDR.

2.3 Viral Delivery

In various human trials, viral vectors have emerged as safe and effective delivery vehicles for clinical gene therapy (Kotterman et al. 2015). Accordingly, viruses were also used to design vectors encoding shRNAs directed against a disease-associated target mRNA, including the ABC-transporter-specific transcripts. For example, adenoviruses encoding anti-ABCB1 shRNAs demonstrated the high potential of this strategy in complete reversal of the multidrug-resistant phenotype in different cancer models in vitro and in vivo (Kaszubiak et al. 2007; Ahn et al. 2010). Likewise, lentiviral vectors derived from HIV-1 demonstrated an efficient downregulation of ABCB1 expression and a successful reversal of the multidrug-resistant phenotype (Ye et al. 2009).

2.4 Bacterial Delivery

In particular for gene therapeutic treatment of bowel-associated diseases, nonpathogenic invasive Escherichia coli strains have been developed (Lage and Fruehauf 2011; Ahmed et al. 2015). In this concept, DNA sequences encoding a therapeutic nucleic acid such as a shRNA directed against a specific molecule are transferred to the target cell by bacteria. Two different steps are required for bacteria to act as delivery systems for therapeutic nucleic acids into mammalian cells: (i) internalization of the microorganisms into the host cell by endocytosis, followed by (ii) escape of the therapeutic bacteria or their therapeutic nucleic acid molecules from the endocytosis vesicle to the cytosol of the target cell. For this approach, Escherichia coli were equipped with a plasmid containing sequences that encode two different proteins that can mediate these two steps. The first protein is invasin of *Yersinia pseudotuberculosis*. Invasin is localized on the bacterial surface and is able to bind to a subset of beta-1-integrins embedded in the cell membranes of mammalian cells including cancer cells. By this binding, the selective uptake by endocytosis of the bacteria by the mammalian host cell is enabled. Subsequent to internalization, *Escherichia coli* are located in a lysosomal endocytosis vesicle where lysis of the microorganisms occurs. Among the various bacterial proteins released into the phagosomal vesicle, lumen is the second protein necessary for therapeutic bacterial delivery, listeriolysin O (LLO) from *Listeria monocytogenes*. This protein is a pore-forming toxin. The cytoplasmic contents of invasive *Escherichia coli*, including therapeutic nucleic acids or proteins, can then escape into the cytosol of the mammalian host cell through the LLO-generated pores. Consequently, this concept was successfully applied for bacteria-mediated delivery of therapeutic molecules in vitro as well as in vivo (Critchley et al. 2004).

By the application of this technology to multidrug-resistant cancer cells, the expression of ABCB1 and the corresponding drug resistance level could be decreased to approximately 50 % of the initial value (Krühn et al. 2009). The technique was not as effective as alternative strategies such as adenoviruses but showed a gentle direct delivery strategy for treatment of multidrug-resistant carcinoma cells derived from gastrointestinal tissues.

2.5 Delivery by Jet-Injection

As discussed, the efficient delivery of RNAi effectors represents the major problem for successful clinical application. In this context, the transfer of naked RNAi-triggering molecules represents an additional alternative to viral, bacterial, and liposomal gene transfer technologies which were described. Various in vitro and in vivo procedures, such as simple needle injection, particle bombardment, in vivo electroporation, or jet-injection, are employed to deliver naked RNAi-mediating nucleic acids into the desired cells or tissues (Walther et al. 2010). These techniques have numerous advantages, such as avoidance of utilization of recombinant viral particles, modified bacterial organisms, reduced or no immunostimulatory potential, and no toxicity.

Among different technologies, jet-injection has gained increasing acceptance, since this technique allows transfer into different tissues with deeper penetration of naked nucleic acids. The jet-injection technology is based on jets of small volumes, which are ejected with high velocity and generate the force to deeply penetrate the targeted tissues and to transfect the affected area. Jet-injection generates broad areas of RNAi effector encoding transgene expression within the jet-injected tissue. The in vivo application of this technology does not induce tissue damage or significant inflammatory reactions at jet-injection sites (Walther et al. 2001).

The technology was successfully applied for reversal of ABCB1-mediated multidrug resistance in cancer cell lines as well as in human cancer xenograft-bearing mice (Stein et al. 2008). Anti-ABCB1 shRNA encoding plasmid vectors decreased the ABCB1 mRNA expression level by more than 90 %. The corresponding transporter protein was no longer detectable in the tumors. By two jet injections of anti-ABCB1 shRNA vectors into the tumors, combined with two intravenous administrations of the cytotoxic drug doxorubicin, were sufficient to achieve complete reversal of the multidrug-resistant phenotype in the tumor xenografts.

3 Conclusion

Although in recent years progress has been made in the development of new gene therapeutic strategies, delivery is still the main hurdle for successful design of gene therapeutic protocols including targeting ABC-transporters for overcoming multidrug resistance. New or improved technologies including RNAi- and CRISPR/Cas9-based approaches may use the long experience obtained with different delivery strategies in the past. Also in future, scientists and clinicians will make assiduous efforts in the development of improved delivery strategies for gene therapeutic agents to target drug-resistant cancer cells.

References

Ahmed O, Krühn A, Lage H (2015) Delivery of siRNAs to cancer cells via bacteria. Methods Mol Biol 1218:117–129

Ahn SJ, Jeon YH, Lee YJ, Lee YL, Lee SW, Ahn BC, Ha JH, Lee J (2010) Enhanced anti-tumor effects of combined MDR1 RNA interference and human sodium/iodide symporter (NIS) radioiodine gene therapy using an adenoviral system in a colon cancer model. Cancer Gene Ther 17:492–500

Critchley RJ, Jezzard S, Radford KJ, Goussard S, Lemoine NR, Grillot-Courvalin C, Vassaux G (2004) Potential therapeutic applications of recombinant, invasive E. coli. Gene Ther 11: 1224–1233

Elbashir SM, Harborth J, Lendeckel W, Yalcin A, Weber K, Tuschl T (2001) Duplexes of 21-nucleotide RNAs mediate RNA interference in cultured mammalian cells. Nature 411: 494–498

Gao Z, Gao Z, Fields JZ, Boman BM (1999) Tumor-specific expression of anti-mdr1 ribozyme selectively restores chemosensitivity in multidrug-resistant colon-adenocarcinoma cells. Int J Cancer 82:346–352

Gilbert LA, Larson MH, Morsut L, Liu Z, Brar GA, Torres SE, Stern-Ginossar N, Brandman O, Whitehead EH, Doudna JA, Lim WA, Weissman JS, Qi LS (2013) CRISPR-mediated modular RNA-guided regulation of transcription in eukaryotes. Cell 154:442–451

Holm PS, Scanlon KJ, Dietel M (1994) Reversion of multidrug resistance in the P-glycoprotein-positive human pancreatic cell line (EPP85-181RDB) by introduction of a hammerhead ribozyme. Br J Cancer 70:239–243

Juliano RL, Ling V (1976) A surface glycoprotein modulating drug permeability in Chinese hamster ovary cell mutants. Biochim Biophys Acta 455:152–162

Kang H, DeLong R, Fisher MH, Juliano RL (2005) Tat-conjugated PAMAM dendrimers as delivery agents for antisense and siRNA oligonucleotides. Pharm Res 22:2099–2106

Kaszubiak A, Holm PS, Lage H (2007) Overcoming the classical multidrug resistance phenotype by adenoviral delivery of anti-MDR1 short hairpin RNAs and ribozymes. Int J Oncol 31: 419–430

Kennedy EM, Kornepati AV, Goldstein M, Bogerd HP, Poling BC, Whisnant AW, Kastan MB, Cullen BR (2014) Inactivation of the human papillomavirus E6 or E7 gene in cervical carcinoma cells by using a bacterial CRISPR/Cas RNA-guided endonuclease. J Virol 88:11965–11972

Kobayashi H, Dorai T, Holland JF, Ohnuma T (1994) Reversal of drug sensitivity in multidrug-resistant tumor cells by an MDR1 (PGY1) ribozyme. Cancer Res 54:1271–1275

Kotterman MA, Chalberg TW, Schaffer DV (2015) Viral vectors for gene therapy: translational and clinical outlook. Annu Rev Biomed Eng 17:63–89

Kowalski P, Surowiak P, Lage H (2005) Reversal of different drug-resistant phenotypes by an autocatalytic multitarget multiribozyme directed against the transcripts of the ABC transporters MDR1/P-gp, MRP2, and BCRP. Mol Ther 11:508–522

Krühn A, Wang A, Fruehauf JH, Lage H (2009) Delivery of short hairpin RNAs by transkingdom RNA interference modulates the classical ABCB1-mediated multidrug-resistant phenotype of cancer cells. Cell Cycle 8:3349–3354

Lage H (2008) An overview of cancer multidrug resistance: a still unsolved problem. Cell Mol Life Sci 65:3145–3167

Lage H (2009) Therapeutic potential of RNA interference in drug-resistant cancers. Future Oncol 5:169–185

Lage H, Fruehauf JH (2011) Delivery of therapeutic RNA molecules to cancer cells by bacteria. Ther Deliv 2:441–449

Nieth C, Priebsch A, Stege A, Lage H (2003) Modulation of the classical multidrug resistance (MDR) phenotype by RNA interference (RNAi). FEBS Lett 545:144–150

Nourbakhsh M, Jaafari MR, Lage H, Abnous K, Mosaffa F, Badiee A, Behravan J (2015) Nanolipoparticles-mediated MDR1 siRNA delivery reduces doxorubicin resistance in breast cancer cells and silences MDR1 expression in xenograft model of human breast cancer. Iran J Basic Med Sci 18:385–392

Patil YB, Swaminathan SK, Sadhukha T, Ma L, Panyam J (2010) The use of nanoparticle-mediated targeted gene silencing and drug delivery to overcome tumor drug resistance. Biomaterials 31:358–365

Simoff I, Karlgren M, Backlund M, Lindström AC, Gaugaz FZ, Matsson P, Artursson P (2016) Complete knockout of endogenous Mdr1 (Abcb1) in MDCK cells by CRISPR-Cas9. J Pharm Sci 105:1017–1021

Soutschek J, Akinc A, Bramlage B, Charisse K, Constien R, Donoghue M, Elbashir S, Geick A, Hadwiger P, Harborth J, John M, Kesavan V, Lavine G, Pandey RK, Racie T, Rajeev KG, Röhl I, Toudjarska I, Wang G, Wuschko S, Bumcrot D, Koteliansky V, Limmer S, Manoharan M, Vornlocher HP (2004) Therapeutic silencing of an endogenous gene by systemic administration of modified siRNAs. Nature 432:173–178

Stege A, Priebsch A, Nieth C, Lage H (2004) Stable and complete overcoming of MDR1/P-glycoprotein-mediated multidrug resistance in human gastric carcinoma cells by RNA interference. Cancer Gene Ther 11:699–706

Stein U, Walther W, Stege A, Kaszubiak A, Fichtner I, Lage H (2008) Complete in vivo reversal of the multidrug resistance (MDR) phenotype by jet-injection of anti-MDR1 short hairpin RNA-encoding plasmid DNA. Mol Ther 16:178–186

Susa M, Iyer AK, Ryu K, Choy E, Hornicek FJ, Mankin H, Milane L, Amiji MM, Duan Z (2010) Inhibition of ABCB1 (MDR1) expression by an siRNA nanoparticulate delivery system to overcome drug resistance in osteosarcoma. PLoS One 5:e10764

Vasanthakumar G, Ahmed NK (1989) Modulation of drug resistance in a daunorubicin resistant subline with oligonucleoside methylphosphonates. Cancer Commun 1:225–232

Walther W, Stein U, Fichtner I, Malcherek L, Lemm M, Schlag PM (2001) Non-viral in vivo gene delivery into tumors using a novel low volume jet-injection technology. Gene Ther 8:173–180

Walther W, Stein U, Lage H (2010) Jet-injection of short hairpin RNA encoding vectors into tumour cells. Methods Mol Biol 629:123–139

Whitehead KA, Langer R, Anderson DG (2009) Knocking down barriers: advances in siRNA delivery. Nat Rev Drug Discov 8:129–138

Wu H, Hait WN, Yang JM (2003) Small interfering RNA-induced suppression of MDR1 (P-glycoprotein) restores sensitivity to multidrug-resistant cancer cells. Cancer Res 63: 1515–1519

Xu H, Li Z, Si J (2014) Nanocarriers in gene therapy: a review. J Biomed Nanotechnol 10: 3483–3507

Yang X, Iyer AK, Singh A, Milane L, Choy E, Hornicek FJ, Amiji MM, Duan Z (2015) Cluster of differentiation 44 targeted hyaluronic acid based nanoparticles for MDR1 siRNA delivery to overcome drug resistance in ovarian cancer. Pharm Res 32:2097–2109

Ye X, Liu T, Gong Y, Zheng B, Meng W, Leng Y (2009) Lentivirus-mediated RNA interference reversing the drug-resistance in MDR1 single-factor resistant cell line K562/MDR1. Leuk Res 33:1114–1119

Yin Q, Shen J, Chen L, Zhang Z, Gu W, Li Y (2012) Overcoming multidrug resistance by co-delivery of Mdr-1 and survivin-targeting RNA with reduction-responsible cationic poly (β-amino esters). Biomaterials 33:6495–6506

Zhao P, Wang H, Gao H, Li C, Zhang Y (2013) Reversal of multidrug resistance by magnetic chitosan-Fe_3O_4 nanoparticle-encapsulated MDR_1 siRNA in glioblastoma cell line. Neurol Res 35:821–828

Bacterial Toxins for Oncoleaking Suicidal Cancer Gene Therapy

Jessica Pahle and Wolfgang Walther

Abstract

For suicide gene therapy, initially prodrug-converting enzymes (gene-directed enzyme-producing therapy, GDEPT) were employed to intracellularly metabolize non-toxic prodrugs into toxic compounds, leading to the effective suicidal killing of the transfected tumor cells. In this regard, the suicide gene therapy has demonstrated its potential for efficient tumor eradication. Numerous suicide genes of viral or bacterial origin were isolated, characterized, and extensively tested in vitro and in vivo, demonstrating their therapeutic potential even in clinical trials to treat cancers of different entities. Apart from this, growing efforts are made to generate more targeted and more effective suicide gene systems for cancer gene therapy. In this regard, bacterial toxins are an alternative to the classical GDEPT strategy, which add to the broad spectrum of different suicide approaches. In this context, lytic bacterial toxins, such as streptolysin O (SLO) or the claudin-targeted *Clostridium perfringens* enterotoxin (CPE) represent attractive new types of suicide oncoleaking genes. They permit as pore-forming proteins rapid and also selective toxicity toward a broad range of cancers. In this chapter, we describe the generation and use of SLO as well as of CPE-based gene therapies for the effective tumor cell eradication as promising, novel suicide gene approach particularly for treatment of therapy refractory tumors.

Keywords

Cancer gene therapy · Suicide gene therapy · Bacterial toxin · Solid tumors

J. Pahle · W. Walther (✉)
Experimental and Clinical Research Center, Charité University Medicine Berlin and Max-Delbrück-Center for Molecular Medicine, Robert-Rössle-Str. 10, 13125 Berlin, Germany
e-mail: wowalt@mdc-berlin.de

W. Walther (ed.), *Current Strategies in Cancer Gene Therapy*,
Recent Results in Cancer Research 209, DOI 10.1007/978-3-319-42934-2_7

1 Introduction

Finding novel and efficient therapies that target malignancies is still important as the incidence of cancer diseases is constantly increasing. Conventional treatment modalities for cancer such as surgery, radiation therapy, and chemotherapy, which are usually combined for a better treatment effect, remain the therapeutic backbone of cancer therapy. However, these therapies do have their limitations, mainly caused by tumor heterogeneity and development of therapy refractory tumor cell populations. During the last decades, anticancer therapy has been continuously improved to overcome these drawbacks, but problems with adverse effects and drug resistance still constitute a main obstacle for successful cancer treatment. Therefore, alternative treatment options are urgently required to efficiently target and eradicate tumors.

Cancer gene therapy represents one such promising strategy, an approach where selective tumor cell killing and tumor growth inhibition can be achieved by introducing foreign nucleic acid (DNA or RNA) as therapeutic agent to tumor cells (Walther and Stein 1999). Genetic therapy can be approached from different directions, such as insertion of a normal gene into cancer cells to replace a mutated or altered gene (Lu et al. 2012; Senzer et al. 2013), selective eradication of tumor cells by suicide mechanisms, induced apoptosis using additive gene insertion (Di Stasi et al. 2011; Zarogoulidis et al. 2013), gene suppression by intervention of gene transcription and translation using, e.g., antisense-oligonucleotides (ASO) (Moulder et al. 2008; Fidias et al. 2009), micro-RNA (miRNA) (Croce 2009) or small interfering double-stranded RNA (siRNA) (Santel et al. 2010; Strumberg et al. 2012). Furthermore, many approaches involve inoculation of immune cells (namely engineered T cells) for immunotherapy. These cells are specifically modified to either replace the immune system to enhance the anti-tumoral response or to boost the patient's own immune system to efficiently kill cancer cells (Kantoff et al. 2010; Sharpe and Mount 2015).

Gene transfer technology comprises a diverse set of therapeutic options and provides promising frontiers for treatment. During the last decades, a broad variety of viral and non-viral vectors have been developed (Gillet et al. 2009). In this regard, replicating and non-replicating viral vectors were improved using retroviral or DNA-virus technology platforms (e.g., lentivirus, adenovirus, AAV, Herpes simplex virus) to increase transfer efficiencies and to improve vector targeting and transgene expression complemented with transcriptional targeting or conditional gene (Walther and Stein 2000). Non-viral systems have entered a new level of quality represented by novel vector types (e.g., minicircle, miniplasmid, dumbbell-shaped minimalistic vectors, sleeping-beauty), transfer technologies including nanoparticles/lipofection and physical technologies (e.g., sonoporation, electroporation, particle bombardment/gene-gun, jet injection). One basic obstacle in cancer gene therapy is the specific targeting directly to a solid tumor. Since particularly in its advanced stages cancer is a metastasizing disease, systemic gene delivery is still one major challenge in cancer gene therapy. Insufficient selectivity and transfer efficiency especially for clinical applications are limiting factors for successful gene therapy and demand improvements in targeting of vector delivery, transgene transcription, and/or translation. In this context, local gene therapy of cancer for local control of the disease is still of some attractiveness and about 20 % of all clinical cancer gene therapy trials are performed as local viral or non-viral gene transfer (Walther et al. 2011b).

Apart from the development of improved transfer technologies, an appropriate therapeutic gene is decisive for a successful cancer treatment. The choice of the respective and most suited gene is often determined by the specific gene therapeutic strategy used for cancer treatment, such as immunogene therapy, suicide gene therapy, gene correction therapy, or gene suppression therapy.

Since long time of the evolution of cancer gene therapy bacterial toxins have complemented the list of therapeutic genes and are attractive candidates as they have demonstrated efficient cell killing capacity in several in vitro and in vivo studies and have shown their potential for effective cancer treatment (Richardson et al. 1999). In this chapter, we will focus on the bacterial toxin-based suicide gene therapy, which is currently gaining increasing attention as treatment option.

2 Suicide Gene Therapy for Cancer Treatment

The major application of suicide gene therapy is focused on treatment of cancer. For this, initially different so-called prodrug-converting enzymes (gene-directed enzyme-producing therapy, GDEPT) of bacterial or viral origin were used for expression in tumor cells, which convert non-toxic prodrugs into toxic metabolites to kill tumor cells and neighboring cells (bystander effect). Most prominent members of these suicide genes are still the cytosine deaminase (CD), Herpes simplex virus thymidine kinase (HSV-tk), cytochrome P450-2B1, and nitroreductase and variants thereof. The CD- and HSV-tk-expressing vectors have long entered clinical phases I and II (Zarogoulidis et al. 2013). Recent developments for these classical suicide genes are aiming at their optimization via mutated variants or fusion proteins for more efficient generation of the toxic metabolites. The term suicide gene therapy has meanwhile broadened toward the delivery of genes that are either directly toxic or pro-apoptotic (Fig. 1).

Even though the ability to kill cancer cells is powerful, there are two major drawbacks of this enzyme-prodrug system: the mentioned bystander effect, which can cause unwanted side effects and a reduced effectiveness in slow-dividing cancer cells. As alternative, suicide gene therapy based on apoptotic genes, such as p53, Bax, or FasL, has been extensively studied but also revealed limitations as cancer cells develop resistance to apoptosis induction (Reed 2002; Igney and Krammer 2002).

Therefore, novel suicide gene therapeutics such as bacterial toxins came into focus, which can overcome the obstacles of resistance and proliferation dependence of the classical suicidal systems.

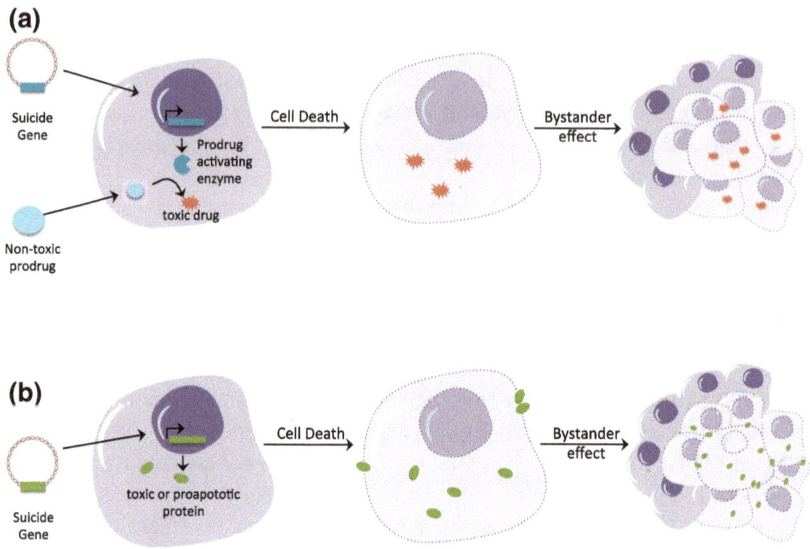

Fig. 1 Targeted killing of cancer cells by using suicide gene therapy. **a** This approach involves the transfer of a therapeutic gene encoding a prodrug-activating enzyme into tumor cells followed by treatment with a specific prodrug. The expression of the therapeutic gene (prodrug-activating enzyme) enables the conversion of the inactive non-toxic prodrug into an active cytotoxic drug. Toxic metabolites can then pass to neighboring cancer cells causing cell killing via the bystander effect. **b** Direct cell killing is also possible if the inserted gene is expressed to produce a toxin-inducing cytotoxicity. As the transfected cells undergo cell death, the expressed toxin can affect neighboring non-transfected cells

3 Bacterial Toxins in Cancer Therapy

The concept of using bacterial toxins as anticancer agents is actually not new as their therapeutic potential was recognized and explored almost 100 years ago (Richardson et al. 1999; Strebhardt and Ullrich 2008). Meanwhile, a continuously growing number of promising experimental in vitro and in vivo studies, using bacterial toxins for cancer treatment, has been published, which reveal their capability of effective cell killing (McCarthy 2006; Patyar et al. 2010; Felgner et al. 2016). In the last decades, the processing and manipulation of toxic bacterial proteins, such as diphtheria toxin, streptolysin O, or clostridium perfringens enterotoxin, and their encoding genes were facilitated, leading to the establishment of "toxin-based therapy" for cancer treatment introducing novel features to suicide gene therapy such as rapid and quite effective pore-forming cell lysis as novel oncoleaking strategy.

3.1 Diphtheria Toxin

One prominent bacterial toxin, which has been extensively used for therapeutic approaches including gene therapies, is the diphtheria toxin (DT). The DT, a 62-kDa exotoxin, secreted by pathogenic strains of *Corynebacterium diphtheria*, binds to the heparin-binding epidermal growth factor precursor (HB-EGF) on the cell surface (Louie et al. 1997). DT consists of 535 amino acids and belongs to the group of AB toxins as it can be cleaved into 2 major fragments (DTA and DTB). The fragment DTB mediates cell entry by binding to a surface receptors and subsequent translocation into cytoplasm by undergoing endocytosis. By contrast, DTA is responsible for the cytotoxic enzymatic activity and inactivates the ADP-ribosylation of elongation factor 2 (EF2), causing inhibition of protein syntheses and cell death (Thorburn et al. 2004; Deng and Barbieri 2008). It is known that the delivery of a single molecule of the catalytic DTA is sufficient to kill a cell, but it is not able to enter a neighboring cell in the absence of DTB (Yamaizumi et al. 1978) (Fig. 2).

3.1.1 DT-Based Suicide Gene Therapy

As mentioned above, DTA is not able to enter a neighboring cell in the absence of DTB. Therefore, it only specifically kills the actual targeted cell, restricting its toxicity. These features of high therapeutic potency, the locally restricted toxic effect, the additional advantages of the evasion of anti-DT immunity, as it is endogenously expressed within the tumor, and the absence of cellular resistance to the toxin supports the great potential of DT-A as gene therapeutic agent.

Nevertheless, this potent bacterial toxin requires efficient and reliable selective targeting, mainly to avoid any unintended side effects on normal cells, which is an essential requirement for the use of the toxin in cancer gene therapy. Several attempts to limit the toxicity of DTA by using modified metallothionein promoter (Maxwell et al. 1986) or by replacement of the wild type DTA sequence with attenuated mutant variants of DTA (Maxwell et al. 1987) were still not able to generate targeted tumor cell killing. To minimize damage to healthy tissue, a specific targeting mechanism was an essential requirement to ensure further use of the toxin.

In the last decades, tissue- and tumor-specific promoter elements were identified, which are critically important for more effective and transcriptionally targeted application of gene therapy (Haviv and Blackwell 2001; Dorer and Nettelbeck 2009). With this knowledge, transcriptional targeting, a method based on positioning the therapeutic gene (e.g., suicide gene) under the transcriptional regulation of a promoter which is specifically or preferentially activated in targeted tumor tissue, was developed (Fukazawa et al. 2004; Saukkonen and Hemminki 2004; Danda et al. 2013). Until today, numerous tissue-specific promoters have been cloned, molecularly characterized, and applied for the controlled DTA expression in different cancer entities.

One example of such promoter is originated from the human H19 RNA gene that is highly expressed in a wide range of cancers and is important for cell proliferation,

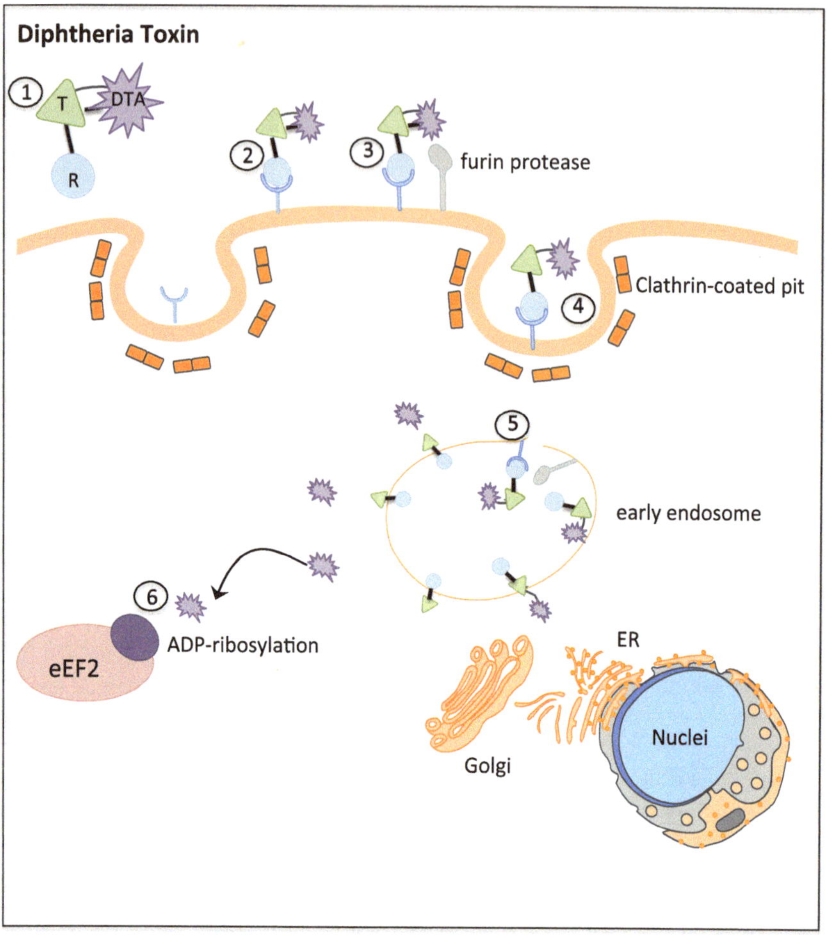

Fig. 2 Mechanism of action of diphtheria toxin. *1* The secreted toxin consists of three functional domains: the N-terminal catalytic domain (DTA), the translocation domain (T), which is bridged by a disulfide bond to the receptor-binding domain (R). *2* DT binds its receptor (heparin-binding epidermal growth factor precursor). *3* The cell surface furin protease cleaves the polypeptide chain between the C and T domains. *4* The toxin-receptor complex is internalized into clathrin-coated pit. *5* Inside the early endosome, furin protease cleaves toxin molecules and T domain undergoes conformational change, inserts into endosome membrane and forms a channel, which leads to translocation of catalytic domain into the cytoplasm, followed by reduction of the disulfide bond. *6* DTA inactivates eukariotic translation elongation factor 2 (eEF2) by ADP-ribosylation, causing inhibition of translation and consequently cell death

genetic instability, vascular angiogenesis, multiple drug resistance, metastasis as well as secondary tumor progression and dissemination (Matouk et al. 2013). Mizrahi et al. reported the use of then H19 gene promoter to drive the targeted expression of DTA in ovarian cancer and demonstrated significant tumor growth inhibition of ovarian cancer xenograft-bearing mice after intratumoral injection of DTA-H19 (Mizrahi et al. 2009). This great potential has been further confirmed in a variety of tumor entities, such as pancreatic cancer (Scaiewicz et al. 2010; Sorin et al. 2012), colon adenocarcinoma (Sorin et al. 2011), or primary lung cancer (Hasenpusch et al. 2011). Thus, DTA-H19 became a "multi-potent vector" (Smaldone and Davies 2010; Amit and Hochberg 2012; Amit et al. 2013) and has entered multiple clinical studies. A phase I and II clinical trial in patients with invasive bladder cancers, receiving intravesical DTA-H19 (namely BC-819) revealed partial and complete response rates as well as prevention of tumor recurrence in two-thirds of treated patients (Gofrit et al. 2014).

Another very recent example for transcriptionally targeted therapy of DT was shown by Tholey et al. They generated DNA-vector constructs with either the pancreatic cancer-specific mesothelin (MSLN) or Mucin 1 (MUC1) promoter linked to DTA coding sequence and combined it with a highly efficient and biodegradable polymer to deliver the vector DNA to pancreatic cancer cells (Tholey et al. 2015). MSLN and MUC1 gene promoters represent promising transcriptional control elements, as they are active at low level in normal cells and highly active a diversity of tumor types, particularly in pancreatic cancer cells, mainly in the most aggressive form that are typically resistant to conventional therapy (Singh and Bandyopadhyay 2007; Showalter et al. 2008; Winter et al. 2012). With this knowledge on promoter activities, MSLN and MUC1 promoter-driven DTA constructs were generated, demonstrating its specific and selective activity as it preferentially kills MSLN/MUC1-expressing pancreatic cancer cells in vitro. A further analysis of matched primary and metastatic tumors in patients showed the great potential of MUC1-targeted therapy as targeting strategy, since this expression is observed consistently in primary tumors and metastasis.

3.2 Streptolysin O

Apart from the strategy of, e.g., of intervention in protein translation by bacterial toxin like DTA, the approach of cell lysis by pore-forming toxins is of attractiveness to eradicate tumor cells. Particularly in light of additional immunostimulation, tumor cell lysis might add to tumor therapy as it deliberates tumor antigens, which could in turn contribute to the activation of the patient's immune response against the tumor. One such pore-forming toxin is streptolysin O (SLO). SLO is a 62-kDa toxin secreted by many strains of Streptococcus bacteria and belongs to the family of pore-forming toxins called cholesterol-dependent cytolysins (CDCs) (Bhakdi et al. 1996). SLO consists of four domains D1–D4, which are rich in β-sheet proportions. The most important protein domains are D3 and D4, as domain D3 provides the transmembrane spanning regions for the toxin and domain D4 directly interacts with cholesterol of the cell membranes. After specifically binding to membrane cholesterols, SLO monomers oligomerize to form homotypic aggregates, which insert into membrane to form a large pore whose diameters can reach up to 35 nm (Shatursky et al. 1999; Sierig et al. 2003) (Fig. 3a).

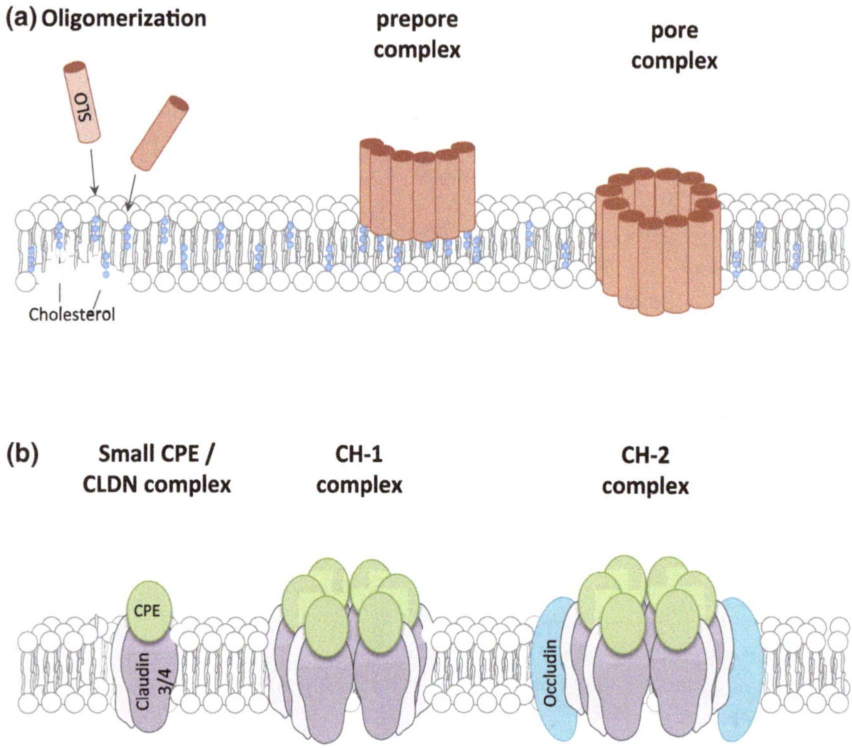

Fig. 3 **a** The mechanism of SLO action. SLO binds specifically to membrane cholesterol and oligomerizes to create a ring structure, which contains 45–50 units and inserts into the membrane to create a large pore, leading to loss of balance between in- and effluxes across the cell membrane. This pore formation further induces cytolysis. **b** The mechanism of CPE binding and mediated cytotoxicity. CPE binds directly to its receptor, preferably claudin-3 or claudin-4, at the plasma membrane of intestinal epithelium. The small CPE/claudin complexes may also include other claudins, e.g., claudin-1, via an indirect interaction. Six small complexes oligomerize to form a large hexameric complex (CH-1), which increases permeability of the cell membrane. CH-1 complexes eventually incorporate occluding, resulting in an even larger complex, namely CH-2, which disrupts epithelial tight junctions resulting in a breakdown of colloid-osmotic equilibrium of affected cells. In consequence, cells undergo cell death by lysis

3.2.1 SLO-Mediated Cytolytic Suicide Gene Therapy

While recombinant SLO protein has been used in several studies for its pore-forming properties, Yang et al. thought of exploiting this particular property of SLO to kill malignant tumor cells and to take the advantage to overcome the anti-apoptotic resistance of cancer cells as well proliferation rate dependence (Yang et al. 2006). Most bacterial toxins, such as diphtheria toxin or pseudomonas exotoxin, tested so far in suicide gene therapy acted “inside” the targeted tumor cell (Martín et al. 2000; Kawakami et al. 2001). Conversely, pore-forming toxins are known to act at the cell membrane and have formerly been used as immunotoxins or recombinant proteins for anticancer treatment. In the study of Yang et al., a conventional plasmid expression vector carrying the SLO gene was used in a liposome-mediated transfection system. Initially, HEK293T cells (human embryonic kidney fibroblasts) were transiently transfected with the SLO vector, leading to cell death caused by cell membrane permeabilization and disintegration. SLO secreted by bacteria usually creates large pores in target cell membrane, allowing large molecules to pass through. To determine whether the observed cytotoxicity in SLO transfected cells was caused by pore formation of expressed SLO lactate dehydrogenase (LDH) release, caspase activity was measured and cells were monitored under electron microscopy. High level of LDH but no caspase activation was observed, indicating that SLO protein expressed within HEK cells induces necrosis. In further studies, they extended their approach by developing an adenoviral expression vector as high-efficiency gene transfer system, which significantly reduced cell viability in several human cancer cell lines (cervical carcinoma cells, C33; lung carcinoma cells, A549; breast cancer cells, MCF-7; and prostate cancer cells, Hep3B). After SLO gene transfer, significant anti-tumoral activity by SLO-mediated cytotoxicity was observed in treated CA33 xenograft-bearing mice.

This study demonstrated the successful use of the SLO gene as anticancer agent in vitro and more importantly in vivo. However, these studies reveal limitations, as the use is limited to local treatment otherwise massive unwanted side effects could occur, since cholesterol is certainly also present in cell membranes of healthy normal cells. Therefore, further modifications like attachment of rather tumor-specific promoters upstream the SLO gene or changing adenoviral fiber proteins, which bind to specific tumor cell surface proteins, are required.

3.3 Clostridium Perfringens Enterotoxin

Another promising pore-forming bacterial toxin for the suicide gene therapy is the clostridium perfringens enterotoxin, which is produced by the anaerobic gram-positive bacterium *Clostridium perfringens* and mainly associated with food poisoning (Minton 2003; Johnson 1999). This 35-kDA single protein contains 319 amino acids with a unique primary sequence. CPE is a two-domain protein that consists of (1) C-terminal receptor-binding domain (amino acid residues 184-319), which recognizes and binds to certain members of the claudin family and an N-terminal domain that is involved in oligomerization and pore formation (Kitadokoro et al. 2011; Briggs et al. 2011).

The C-terminal fragment of CPE (c-CPE) reveals a high-affinity binding to its receptors, for example, claudin-3 or claudin-4; however, it is not able to initiate or form pores (Hanna et al. 1991). The N-terminal residues 80–160 also referred to as TM1 region consist of hydrophilic and hydrophobic amino acids, which resemble the β-loops, which then mediate membrane insertion and pore formation. The mechanism of action of CPE is initiated by the binding to its natural receptors, the transmembrane proteins claudin. In particular, claudin-3, claudin-4, claudin-6, claudin-6, and claudin-14 are proven CPE receptors (Katahira et al. 1997; Fujita et al. 2000; Lal-Nag et al. 2012; Shrestha and McClane 2013; Shrestha et al. 2016).

The claudin family consists of at least 27 proteins that are essential for tight junction formation in epithelial and endothelial cells. They also play an important role in controlling paracellular transport and maintenance of cell polarity (Gumbiner 1987). Claudins are comprised of four transmembrane domains; a C-terminal cytoplasmic tail; and two extracellular loops, ECL1 and ECL2 (Günzel and Fromm 2012). The binding of CPE to its claudin receptor triggers the formation of a "small complex" (90 kDa), containing CPE and the receptor (Tsukita and Furuse 2000; Smedley et al. 2007). This small complex by itself is not able to mediate cytoxicity, but several small complexes interact and oligomerize to a prepore on the membrane surface, which results in a 450-kDa "large complex"—named CH-1 complex (Robertson et al. 2007). The CH-1 complex that comprises a CPE hexamer and claudins subsequently forms a pore into the membrane, causing membrane permeability alterations, and permits a calcium influx, inducing cell death (Matsuda and Sugimoto 1979; Freedman et al. 2016). The morphological damage leads to exposure of the basolateral cell surface, allowing additional binding of the toxin to form an even larger ~600-kDa complex, known as CH-2, which consists of claudins as well as occludin (Singh et al. 2000) (Fig. 3b).

So far it is known that high CPE concentration causes formation of many pores, leading to a massive calcium influx and consequently to necrotic cell death, whereas low CPE concentration results in formation of low number of pores, rather causing apoptosis (Chakrabarti et al. 2003).

3.3.1 CPE-Based Oncoleaking Suicide Gene Therapy

Numerous studies have shown that certain cancer entities, particularly epithelial cancers, such as colon, breast, prostate, ovarian, and pancreatic cancer, possess a high expression of claudin-3 and/or claudin-4 (Rangel et al. 2003; Hewitt et al. 2006; Santin et al. 2007; Takala et al. 2007; Kominsky et al. 2007; Saeki et al. 2009; Neesse et al. 2012; Lu et al. 2013). Due to this fact, considerable effort has been made to develop a CPE-based approach for cancer therapy and its potential clinical benefit in targeting claudin-3- and claudin-4-expressing tumors has been evaluated. The application of recombinant CPE protein demonstrated a dose-dependent cell killing of claudin-3 and claudin-4-overexpressing pancreatic, breast or colon cancer cells in vitro and in vivo (Litkouhi et al. 2007; Saeki et al. 2009; Gao and McClane 2012; Kojima et al. 2012). In addition to that, the intratumoral application in tumor bearing mice did not induce unwanted toxin-associated side effects. However, the use of recombinant CPE protein requires repeated application of the toxin to achieve significant therapeutic effect (Michl et al. 2001; Kominsky et al. 2004). Alternatively, the gene transfer of a CPE-expressing vector could be sufficient to significantly prolong toxin availability and improve intratumoral dispersion and subsequently amplify the cytotoxic effect.

Based on this idea, we established an eukaryotic translation optimized CPE vector (optCPE), which combines both target specificity and efficient cytotoxicity (Walther et al. 2011a). The intracellular CPE expression and accumulation after gene transfer led to effective eradication of claudin-3 and claudin-4 high-expressing cells, such as the mammary carcinoma cell line MCF-7 or the human pancreatic cancer cells Panc1, whereas claudin-negative cells like the melanoma cell line Sk-Mel5 remained unaffected. This study further demonstrated that even though CPE is produced inside the transfected cell, its outside action of binding to the claudins and mediating pore formation and cell lysis is not hampered.

More importantly, it was shown that non-viral intratumoral gene transfer of CPE-expressing plasmid-vector does induce extensive tumor necrosis in HCT116 human colon carcinoma and in MCF-7 human mammary carcinoma xenotransplanted mice. This was associated with significant reduction in tumor growth and showed improved efficacy over treatments with the recombinant CPE, which was well tolerated by the animals.

In our very recent study, we employed the optCPE gene therapy to selectively eradicate claudin-3 and claudin-4-expressing pancreatic carcinomas and demonstrated again the successful use of this suicide gene therapy approach as CPE expression permitted rapid tumor destruction in vitro (Pahle et al. 2015).

In both studies, we observed the presence of released biological active CPE in the media of all transfected cells (claudin-positive and claudin-negative cells), suggesting a cytotoxicity-independent deliberation of CPE, which further supports the concept of bystander effect that strongly contributes to the efficiency of this gene therapy approach (Fig. 1b).

For the improved and more effective use of the toxin, the mode of cell death, induced by transfected CPE is of interest. The analysis on cell death mechanism revealed that delayed activation of the caspases 3/7 was induced, indicating rather CPE-mediated necrosis than apoptosis. This was further supported by the dramatic increase of LDH release after CPE transfection and appearance of necrotic cell morphology, such as cell membrane and nuclear rupture. As mentioned above and reported by others, cell death mechanism is dependent on CPE concentration, number of pores generated by CPE and claudin localization (tight junctions, cell membrane, cytoplasm) of targeted cell, which determines accessibility for CPE binding.

Taken together, CPE oncoleaking gene therapy is of great value for the targeted eradication of therapy refractory tumors, which is further improved by the bystander effect of this particular suicide approach.

4 Conclusions

As gene therapy comes of age, it has shown its efficacy for the treatment of cancer diseases reflected by the application of this strategy in clinical trials. In fact, more than 7 % of all gene therapy clinical trials worldwide are employing suicide approaches either as monotherapy or in combination with other, conventional therapies such as chemo- and radiotherapy. Numerous suicidal systems have been established and successfully employed and among them bacterial toxins might experience some thorough re-evaluation as potential tools for more effective and to some extend more targeted gene therapies. In this regard, pore-forming, oncoleaking bacterial toxins such as SLO or CPE hold promise for the efficient and rapid tumor cell killing. In particular CPE action is associated with selective tumor cell killing properties targeting the claudin-3 and claudin-4 tight junction proteins, which are often deregulated in epithelial cancers. As shown for meanwhile classical suicidal systems (e.g., CD, HSV-tk), bacterial toxins like CPE do also possess the feature of bystander effect, which is important if not essential for effective in vivo use of this suicide gene therapeutic. These initial studies for the use of bacterial toxins for oncoleaking suicide therapies might further promote the directed search for novel, similarly or even more effective and tumor-targeted toxins that can potentially be used for cancer gene therapy.

References

Amit D, Hochberg A (2012) Development of targeted therapy for a broad spectrum of cancers (pancreatic cancer, ovarian cancer, glioblastoma and HCC) mediated by a double promoter plasmid expressing diphtheria toxin under the control of H19 and IGF2-P4 regulatory sequences. Int J Clin Exp Med 5:296–305

Amit D, Tamir S, Hochberg A (2013) Development of targeted therapy for a broad spectrum of solid tumors mediated by a double promoter plasmid expressing diphtheria toxin under the control of IGF2-P4 and IGF2-P3 regulatory sequences. Int J Clin Exp Med 6:110–118. doi:10.1186/1479-5876-8-134

Bhakdi S, Bayley H, Valeva A et al (1996) Staphylococcal alpha-toxin, streptolysin-O, and Escherichia coli hemolysin: prototypes of pore-forming bacterial cytolysins. Arch Microbiol 165:73–79. doi:10.1007/s002030050300

Briggs DC, Naylor CE, Smedley JG et al (2011) Structure of the food-poisoning Clostridium perfringens enterotoxin reveals similarity to the aerolysin-like pore-forming toxins. J Mol Biol 413:138–149. doi:10.1016/j.jmb.2011.07.066

Chakrabarti G, Zhou X, McClane BA (2003) Death pathways activated in CaCo-2 cells by Clostridium perfringens enterotoxin. Infect Immun 71:4260–4270

Croce CM (2009) Causes and consequences of microRNA dysregulation in cancer. Nat Rev Genet 10:704–714. doi:10.1038/nrg2634

Danda R, Krishnan G, Ganapathy K et al (2013) Targeted expression of suicide gene by tissue-specific promoter and microRNA regulation for cancer gene therapy. PLoS ONE 8: e83398. doi:10.1371/journal.pone.0083398

Deng Q, Barbieri JT (2008) Molecular mechanisms of the cytotoxicity of ADP-ribosylating toxins. Annu Rev Microbiol 62:271–288. doi:10.1146/annurev.micro.62.081307.162848

Di Stasi A, Tey S-K, Dotti G et al (2011) Inducible apoptosis as a safety switch for adoptive cell therapy. N Engl J Med 365:1673–1683. doi:10.1056/NEJMoa1106152

Dorer DE, Nettelbeck DM (2009) Targeting cancer by transcriptional control in cancer gene therapy and viral oncolysis. Adv Drug Deliv Rev 61:554–571. doi:10.1016/j.addr.2009.03.013

Felgner S, Kocijancic D, Frahm M, Weiss S (2016) Bacteria in cancer therapy: renaissance of an old concept. Int J Microbiol 2016:1–14. doi:10.1155/2016/8451728

Fidias P, Pennell NA, Boral AL et al (2009) Phase I study of the c-raf-1 antisense oligonucleotide ISIS 5132 in combination with carboplatin and paclitaxel in patients with previously untreated, advanced non-small cell lung cancer. J Thorac Oncol 4:1156–1162. doi:10.1097/JTO.0b013e3181b2793f

Freedman J, Shrestha A, McClane B (2016) Clostridium perfringens Enterotoxin: action, genetics, and translational applications. Toxins (Basel) 8:73. doi:10.3390/toxins8030073

Fujita K, Katahira J, Horiguchi Y et al (2000) Clostridium perfringens enterotoxin binds to the second extracellular loop of claudin-3, a tight junction integral membrane protein. FEBS Lett 476:258–261
Fukazawa T, Maeda Y, Sladek FM, Owen-Schaub LB (2004) Development of a cancer-targeted tissue-specific promoter system. Cancer Res 64:363–369. doi:10.1158/0008-5472.can-03-2507
Gao Z, McClane B a (2012) Use of Clostridium perfringens enterotoxin and the enterotoxin receptor-binding domain (C-CPE) for cancer treatment: opportunities and challenges. J Toxicol 2012:981626. doi:10.1155/2012/981626
Gillet J-P, Macadangdang B, Fathke RL et al (2009) The development of gene therapy: from monogenic recessive disorders to complex diseases such as cancer. Methods Mol Biol Clift NJ 542:5–54
Gofrit ON, Benjamin S, Halachmi S et al (2014) DNA based therapy with diphtheria toxin-A BC-819: a phase 2b marker lesion trial in patients with intermediate risk nonmuscle invasive bladder cancer. J Urol 191:1697–1702. doi:10.1016/j.juro.2013.12.011
Gumbiner B (1987) Structure, biochemistry, and assembly of epithelial tight junctions. Am J Physiol 253:C749–C758
Günzel D, Fromm M (2012) Claudins and other tight junction proteins. Compr Physiol 2:1819–1852. doi:10.1002/cphy.c110045
Hanna PC, Mietzner TA, Schoolnik GK, McClane BA (1991) Localization of the receptor-binding region of Clostridium perfringens enterotoxin utilizing cloned toxin fragments and synthetic peptides. The 30 C-terminal amino acids define a functional binding region. J Biol Chem 266:11037–11043
Hasenpusch G, Pfeifer C, Aneja MK et al (2011) Aerosolized BC-819 inhibits primary but not secondary lung cancer growth. PLoS ONE 6:e20760. doi:10.1371/journal.pone.0020760
Haviv YS, Blackwell J (2001) Transcriptional regulation in cancer gene therapy. Isr Med Assoc J 3:517–522
Hewitt KJ, Agarwal R, Morin PJ (2006) The claudin gene family: expression in normal and neoplastic tissues. BMC Cancer 6:186. doi:10.1186/1471-2407-6-186
Igney FH, Krammer PH (2002) Death and anti-death: tumour resistance to apoptosis. Nat Rev Cancer 2:277–288. doi:10.1038/nrc776
Johnson EA (1999) Clostridial toxins as therapeutic agents: benefits of natur's most toxic proteins. Annu Rev Microbiol 53:551–75. doi:10.1146/annurev.micro.53.1.551
Kantoff PW, Higano CS, Shore ND et al (2010) Sipuleucel-T immunotherapy for castration-resistant prostate cancer. N Engl J Med 363:411–422. doi:10.1056/NEJMoa1001294
Katahira J, Inoue N, Horiguchi Y et al (1997) Molecular cloning and functional characterization of the receptor for Clostridium perfringens enterotoxin. J Cell Biol 136:1239–1247
Kawakami K, Kawakami M, Joshi BH, Puri RK (2001) Interleukin-13 receptor-targeted cancer therapy in an immunodeficient animal model of human head and neck cancer. Cancer Res 61:6194–6200
Kitadokoro K, Nishimura K, Kamitani S et al (2011) Crystal structure of Clostridium perfringens enterotoxin displays features of beta-pore-forming toxins. J Biol Chem 286:19549–19555. doi:10.1074/jbc.M111.228478
Kojima T, Kyuno D, Sawada N (2012) Targeting claudin-4 in human pancreatic cancer. Expert Opin Ther Targets 16:881–887. doi:10.1517/14728222.2012.708340
Kominsky SL, Tyler B, Sosnowski J et al (2007) Clostridium perfringens enterotoxin as a novel-targeted therapeutic for brain metastasis. Cancer Res 67:7977–7982. doi:10.1158/0008-5472.CAN-07-1314
Kominsky SL, Vali M, Korz D et al (2004) Clostridium perfringens enterotoxin elicits rapid and specific cytolysis of breast carcinoma cells mediated through tight junction proteins claudin 3 and 4. Am J Pathol 164:1627–1633
Lal-Nag M, Battis M, Santin a D, Morin PJ (2012) Claudin-6: a novel receptor for CPE-mediated cytotoxicity in ovarian cancer. Oncogenesis 1:e33. doi:10.1038/oncsis.2012.32

Litkouhi B, Kwong J, Lo C-M et al (2007) Claudin-4 overexpression in epithelial ovarian cancer is associated with hypomethylation and is a potential target for modulation of tight junction barrier function using a C-terminal fragment of Clostridium perfringens enterotoxin. Neoplasia 9:304–314

Louie GV, Yang W, Bowman ME, Choe S (1997) Crystal structure of the complex of diphtheria toxin with an extracellular fragment of its receptor. Mol Cell 1:67–78. doi:10.1016/S1097-2765(00)80008-8

Lu C, Stewart DJ, Lee JJ et al (2012) Phase I clinical trial of systemically administered TUSC2 (FUS1)-nanoparticles mediating functional gene transfer in humans. PLoS ONE 7:e34833. doi:10.1371/journal.pone.0034833

Lu Z, Ding L, Lu Q, Chen Y-H (2013) Claudins in intestines: distribution and functional significance in health and diseases. Tissue barriers 1:e24978

Martín V, Cortés ML, de Felipe P et al (2000) Cancer gene therapy by thyroid hormone-mediated expression of toxin genes. Cancer Res 60:3218–3224

Matouk I, Raveh E, Ohana P et al (2013) The increasing complexity of the oncofetal h19 gene locus: functional dissection and therapeutic intervention. Int J Mol Sci 14:4298–4316. doi:10.3390/ijms14024298

Matsuda M, Sugimoto N (1979) Calcium-independent and dependent steps in action of Clostridiumperfringens enterotoxin on HeLa and Vero cells. Biochem Biophys Res Commun 91:629–636. doi:10.1016/0006-291X(79)91568-7

Maxwell F, Maxwell IH, Glode LM (1987) Cloning, sequence determination, and expression in transfected cells of the coding sequence for the tox 176 attenuated diphtheria toxin A chain. Mol Cell Biol 7:1576–1579

Maxwell IH, Maxwell F, Glode LM (1986) Regulated expression of a diphtheria toxin A-chain gene transfected into human cells: possible strategy for inducing cancer cell suicide. Cancer Res 46:4660–4.

McCarthy EF (2006) The toxins of William B. Coley and the treatment of bone and soft-tissue sarcomas. Iowa Orthop J 26:154–158

Michl P, Buchholz M, Rolke M et al (2001) Claudin-4: a new target for pancreatic cancer treatment using Clostridium perfringens enterotoxin. Gastroenterology 121:678–684. doi:10.1053/gast.2001.27124

Minton NP (2003) Clostridia in cancer therapy. Nat Rev Microbiol 1:237–242

Mizrahi A, Czerniak A, Levy T et al (2009) Development of targeted therapy for ovarian cancer mediated by a plasmid expressing diphtheria toxin under the control of H19 regulatory sequences. J Transl Med 7:69. doi:10.1186/1479-5876-7-69

Moulder SL, Symmans WF, Booser DJ et al (2008) Phase I/II study of G3139 (Bcl-2 antisense oligonucleotide) in combination with doxorubicin and docetaxel in breast cancer. Clin Cancer Res 14:7909–7916. doi:10.1158/1078-0432.CCR-08-1104

Neesse a, Griesmann H, Gress TM, Michl P (2012) Claudin-4 as therapeutic target in cancer. Arch Biochem Biophys 524:64–70. doi:10.1016/j.abb.2012.01.009

Pahle J, Aumann J, Kobelt D, Walther W (2015) Oncoleaking: use of the pore-forming clostridium perfringens enterotoxin (CPE) for suicide gene therapy. Methods Mol Biol 1317:69–85. doi:10.1007/978-1-4939-2727-2_5

Patyar S, Joshi R, Byrav DP et al (2010) Bacteria in cancer therapy: a novel experimental strategy. J Biomed Sci 17:21

Rangel LBA, Agarwal R, D'Souza T et al (2003) Tight junction proteins claudin-3 and claudin-4 are frequently overexpressed in ovarian cancer but not in ovarian cystadenomas. Clin Cancer Res 9:2567–2575

Reed JC (2002) Apoptosis-based therapies. Nat Rev Drug Discov 1:111–121. doi:10.1038/nrd726

Richardson MA, Ramirez T, Russell NC, Moye LA (1999) Coley toxins immunotherapy: a retrospective review. Altern Ther Health Med 5:42–47

Robertson SL, Smedley JG, Singh U et al (2007) Compositional and stoichiometric analysis of Clostridium perfringens enterotoxin complexes in Caco-2 cells and claudin 4 fibroblast transfectants. Cell Microbiol 9:2734–2755
Saeki R, Kondoh M, Kakutani H et al (2009) A novel tumor-targeted therapy using a claudin-4-targeting molecule. Mol Pharmacol 76:918–926
Santel A, Aleku M, Röder N et al (2010) Atu027 prevents pulmonary metastasis in experimental and spontaneous mouse metastasis models. Clin Cancer Res 16:5469–5480. doi:10.1158/1078-0432.CCR-10-1994
Santin AD, Bellone S, Siegel ER et al (2007) Overexpression of Clostridium perfringens enterotoxin receptors claudin-3 and claudin-4 in uterine carcinosarcomas. Clin Cancer Res 13:3339–3346
Saukkonen K, Hemminki A (2004) Tissue-specific promoters for cancer gene therapy. Expert Opin Biol Ther 4:683–96
Scaiewicz V, Sorin V, Fellig Y et al (2010) Use of H19 gene regulatory sequences in DNA-based therapy for pancreatic cancer. J Oncol 2010:178174. doi:10.1155/2010/178174
Senzer N, Nemunaitis J, Nemunaitis D et al (2013) Phase I study of a systemically delivered p53 nanoparticle in advanced solid tumors. Mol Ther 21:1096–1103. doi:10.1038/mt.2013.32
Sharpe M, Mount N (2015) Genetically modified T cells in cancer therapy: opportunities and challenges. Dis Model Mech 8:337–350. doi:10.1242/dmm.018036
Shatursky O, Heuck AP, Shepard LA et al (1999) The mechanism of membrane insertion for a cholesterol-dependent cytolysin. Cell 99:293–299. doi:10.1016/S0092-8674(00)81660-8
Showalter S, Huang Y-H, Witkiewicz A et al (2008) Nanoparticulate delivery of diphtheria toxin DNA effectively kills mesothelin expressing pancreatic cancer cells. Cancer Bio Ther 7:1584–1590
Shrestha A, McClane BA (2013) Human claudin-8 and -14 are receptors capable of conveying the cytotoxic effects of Clostridium perfringens enterotoxin. MBio. doi:10.1128/mBio.00594-12
Shrestha A, Uzal FA, McClane BA (2016) The interaction of Clostridium perfringens enterotoxin with receptor claudins. Anaerobe 41:18–26. doi:10.1016/j.anaerobe.2016.04.011
Sierig G, Cywes C, Wessels MR, Ashbaugh CD (2003) Cytotoxic effects of streptolysin o and streptolysin s enhance the virulence of poorly encapsulated group a streptococci. Infect Immun 71:446–455
Singh R, Bandyopadhyay D (2007) MUC1: a target molecule for cancer therapy. Cancer Biol Ther 6:481–486
Singh U, Van Itallie CM, Mitic LL et al (2000) CaCo-2 cells treated with Clostridium perfringens enterotoxin form multiple large complex species, one of which contains the tight junction protein occludin. J Biol Chem 275:18407–18417
Smaldone MC, Davies BJ (2010) BC-819, a plasmid comprising the H19 gene regulatory sequences and diphtheria toxin A, for the potential targeted therapy of cancers. Curr Opin Mol Ther 12:607–616
Smedley JG, Uzal FA, McClane BA (2007) Identification of a prepore large-complex stage in the mechanism of action of Clostridium perfringens enterotoxin. Infect Immun 75:2381–2390
Sorin V, Ohana P, Gallula J et al (2012) H19-promoter-targeted therapy combined with gemcitabine in the treatment of pancreatic cancer. ISRN Oncol 2012:351750. doi:10.5402/2012/351750
Sorin V, Ohana P, Mizrahi A et al (2011) Regional therapy with DTA-H19 vector suppresses growth of colon adenocarcinoma metastases in the rat liver. Int J Oncol 39:1407–1412
Strebhardt K, Ullrich A (2008) Paul Ehrlich's magic bullet concept: 100 years of progress. Nat Rev Cancer 8:473–480. doi:10.1038/nrc2394
Strumberg D, Schultheis B, Traugott U et al (2012) Phase I clinical development of Atu027, a siRNA formulation targeting PKN3 in patients with advanced solid tumors. Int J Clin Pharmacol Ther 50:76–78

Takala H, Saarnio J, Wiik H, Soini Y (2007) Claudins 1, 3, 4, 5 and 7 in esophageal cancer: loss of claudin 3 and 4 expression is associated with metastatic behavior. APMIS Acta Pathol Microbiol Immunol Scand 115:838–847
Tholey RM, Lal S, Jimbo M et al (2015) MUC1 promoter-driven DTA as a targeted therapeutic strategy against pancreatic cancer. Mol Cancer Res 13:439–448. doi:10.1158/1541-7786.MCR-14-0199
Thorburn A, Thorburn J, Frankel AE (2004) Induction of apoptosis by tumor cell-targeted toxins. Apoptosis 9:19–25. doi:10.1023/B:APPT.0000012118.95548.88
Tsukita S, Furuse M (2000) Pores in the wall: claudins constitute tight junction strands containing aqueous pores. J Cell Biol 149:13–16
Walther W, Petkov S, Kuvardina ON et al (2011a) Novel Clostridium perfringens enterotoxin suicide gene therapy for selective treatment of claudin-3- and -4-overexpressing tumors. Gene Ther 19:494–503. doi:10.1038/gt.2011.136
Walther W, Schlag PM, Stein U (2011b) Local gene delivery for therapy of solid tumors. Drug delivery in oncology. Wiley-VCH Verlag GmbH & Co. KGaA, Weinheim, pp 1391–1413
Walther W, Stein U (1999) Therapeutic genes for cancer gene therapy. Mol Biotechnol 13:21–28. doi:10.1385/MB:13:1:21
Walther W, Stein U Walther W, Stein U (2000) Viral vectors for gene transfer: a review of their use in the treatment of human diseases. Drugs 60:249–271. jourlib.org. http://www.jourlib.org/references/5588026. Accessed 30 Sep 2015
Winter JM, Tang LH, Klimstra DS et al (2012) A novel survival-based tissue microarray of pancreatic cancer validates MUC1 and mesothelin as biomarkers. PLoS ONE 7:e40157. doi:10.1371/journal.pone.0040157
Yamaizumi M, Mekada E, Uchida T et al (1978) One molecule of diphtheria toxin fragment a introduced into a cell can kill the cell. Cell 15:245–250. doi:10.1016/0092-8674(78)90099-5
Yang WS, Park S-O, Yoon A-R et al (2006) Suicide cancer gene therapy using pore-forming toxin, streptolysin O. Mol Cancer Ther 5:1610–1619. doi:10.1158/1535-7163.MCT-05-0515
Zarogoulidis P, Darwiche K, Sakkas A et al (2013) Suicide gene therapy for cancer—current strategies. J Genet Syndr gene Ther 9(4pii):16849. doi:10.4172/2157-7412.1000139

Use of Bacteria in Cancer Therapy

Pooja Sarotra and Bikash Medhi

Abstract

Cancer is one of the most dreaded diseases in humans and most common cause of death in twenty-first century. New cancer therapies are urgently required because of the existing pharmacological side effects of the conventional chemotherapy, radiation, or surgery. Newer modalities such as cancer vaccines and biological therapies are proving very helpful in the treatment of cancer along with the conventional therapies. The success of these novel cancer therapies is attributed to their lesser toxicity and the specific killing of the cancer cells. Bacterial therapy for cancer has been recognized a century ago. Live, attenuated, or genetically modified obligate or facultative anaerobic bacterial species exhibit the inherent property of colonizing the tumors and are capable of multiplying selectively inside the tumors, thereby inhibiting cancerous growths. The bacteria and their spores are used in the target specific therapies, delivering the prodrugs and the various proteins to the tumors. Albeit bacterial treatment of cancer is providing new perspective in the treatment of disease, the use of microorganisms to target tumors has certain confinements. The biosafety, genetic instability and the confounded interaction of the bacteria with treatment drugs, requires the more noteworthy consideration regarding the use of this novel treatment in the cancer treatment.

Keywords

Bacterial vectors · Bacterial toxins · Suicide genes · Immunostimulation · Oncolytic therapy · Tumor targeting

P. Sarotra · B. Medhi (✉)
Department of Pharmacology, Post Graduate Institute of Medical Education and Research, Chandigarh 160012, India
e-mail: drbikashus@yahoo.com

W. Walther (ed.), *Current Strategies in Cancer Gene Therapy*,
Recent Results in Cancer Research 209, DOI 10.1007/978-3-319-42934-2_8

1 Background

Cancer can be defined as biomedically complicated group of diseases resulting partly from the mutations of genes that control the cell growth and behavior and partly due to the interactions of cellular stresses and the genetic changes inflicted from specific environmental factors.

Hanahan and Weinberg suggested in 2000 in their famous review "The hallmarks of cancer" human tumors display six common features: self-sufficiency in growth signals, avoidance of programmed cell death (apoptosis), insensitivity to growth-inhibitory signals, infinite growth potential, sustained blood vessel formation (angiogenesis), and tissue invasion and spread to other sites (metastasis). There have been new additions to these features such as chromosome abnormalities, abnormal metabolic pathways, and evasion of the immune system and inflammation Hanahan and Weinberg (2011). Most types of cancer cells eventually outgrow to form a lump or mass called as tumor and the nomenclature of the cancer type is based on the origin of tumor from the respective body part.

Cancer is one of the dreaded diseases of the century killing millions all over the world. It is currently the cause of 12 % of all deaths worldwide. By 2030, it is projected that there will be 26 million new cancer cases and 17 million cancer deaths per year. The management of the disease is different, based on the stages and the origin of the cancer. The conventional therapies such as chemotherapy, surgical resection, targeted therapy, immunotherapy, hormonal therapy, and radiotherapy have been proved to be effective with pharmacological side effects. However, resistant tumors have shown to metastases the organs in the cancer patients and conventional therapies become ineffective. Hence, novel therapies are required that may be supplemented to the conventional therapies or by itself prove to be a cure for the disease.

1.1 History of the Usage of the Bacteria in Cancer

German physicians, Busch and Fehleisen, have used bacteria as an anticancer agent around 150 years ago. They have observed that accidental skin infections (erysipelas) caused by *Streptococcus pyogenes* were able to regress the tumors of patients. Twenty years later, American Physician, William Coley, noticed that the patient diagnosed with neck cancer recovered due to the infection of erysipelas. He conducted experimentation and hence documented the proof that several patients with end-stage cancers exhibited the tumor regression after infecting with killed bacterial species *S. pyogenes* and *Serrati amarcescens*. The earlier success of Coley toxins has paved the current ground for the advances in the bacterial therapy in cancer.

In 1935, Connell observed tumor regression with sterile filtrates having enzymes from *Clostridium histolyticum* in metastatic cancer. Nevertheless, this field was stagnant due to increased deaths by bacterial infections as well as other drawbacks.

The revolution for the utilization of microscopic bacterial organisms was given by Morales, Eidinger, and Bruce. The group has reported fruitful treatment of bladder cancer with Bacillus Calmette–Guérin (BCG) (Patyar et al. 2010).

2 Tumor Targeting Bacteria

Bacterial genomes are very simple. These can be easily manipulated and amplified. The recombinant biology is successful because of the easy proliferation of the bacteria and of low maintenance cost. Certain anaerobic bacteria can grow easily in the oxygen-deprived condition of the tumors. There is an environment of increased vasculature with metabolic by-products and inflammation associated with the tumor growths, and the anaerobes can easily survive such conditions and hence can easily destroy the tumor. An approach to the synthetic biology could be used to enhance target specificity and efficacy with lessened toxicity. Numerous genera of bacteria such as *Salmonella, Escherichia, Clostridium, Bifidobacterium, Caulobacter, Listeria, Proteus,* and *Streptococcus* have been investigated for anticancerous properties over the past century. Some of the bacteria can naturally colonize the tumors with inherent tumor targeting ability. Gram-positive anaerobes, for example *Bifidobacteria* and *Clostridia,* can colonize the oxygen-deficient areas within the necrotic and/or hypoxic areas of tumors, whereas Gram-negative facultative anaerobes, for example *Salmonella*, can invade and grow inside as well as outside the tumors.

Initial experimental studies with the pathogenic species of anaerobic *clostridia* have shown the preferential proliferation within the tumors along with acute toxicity and death of the animals. These studies led to shift the focus on the non-pathogenic *Clostridium* strains despite lesser success in tumor regression. *Clostridium novyi* has exhibited a significant success in reducing the tumor. *C. novyi-NT* has been attenuated after deleting the gene coding for the lethal toxin and has been successfully used for tumor regressions. Recent study by Roberts et al. (2014) has shown that injecting the *C. novyi* spores into the tumors of dogs has demonstrated the tumors shrank or disappeared. The study was extended to the clinical trial showing the disintegration of the tumor.

Frahm et al. (2015) have genetically manipulated the Salmonella as a part of a cancer therapy. They modified the lipopolysaccharide structure (LPS) that induces sepsis and made the bacteria less harmful. The introduction of the arabinose promoter inside the bacteria helped in the effective colonizing of bacteria in the tumors. There was transition of the salmonella that can grow every hour inside the tumor and was able to kill the cancer cells in the mice.

In 2010, Forbes proposed a model of smart bacteria that can specifically target tumors, self-propelling, produce the cytotoxic molecules, steers toward chemo-attractants Forbes (2010). Through the careful tuning of the bacterial phages, Forbes gave the concept of the perfect bacteria or robot factory for the cancer therapy.

3 Expression of Anticancerous Agents

The simple genomes of bacteria can be genetically engineered to express anticancer agents to increase the efficacy. Bacterial vectors display the ability to carry, make, and deliver anticancer agents in the form of drugs, therapeutic DNA, microRNA, shRNA, siRNA, cytotoxic agents, antiangiogenic agents, and specific enzymes that convert prodrugs into anticancer drugs. Bacteria have its own complete complement of the genetic machinery and hence, capable of making and delivering the macromolecules at the specific targets. This phenomenon has been demonstrated envisaging the direct expression of the anti-tumor proteins and transfecting the cancerous cells with eukaryotic expression vectors (Table 1).

In the direct expression, the main anticancer therapies that can be categorized are the expression of the proteins that can kill the tumor cells; expression of cytotoxic agents; expression of antiangiogenic agents; and expression of the enzymes that can catalyze the conversion of the non-functional prodrug to an activated anticancer

Table 1 Bacterial strategies for cancer therapy

Strategies		Genus
Tumoricidal agent	Live, attenuated, genetically engineered	*Salmonella, Escherichia, Clostridium, Bifidobacterium, Caulobacter, Listeria, Proteus, Streptococcus*
Expressing anticancer agents as recombinant bacteria	Cytotoxic: cytolysin A, tNFα, TRAIL, FASL Cytokines: IL-2, IL-12, IL-10 Anti-angiogenic agents: Endostatin Enzymes for prodrugs conversion: Herpes simplex virus thymidine kinase (HSV-TK) with ganciclovir (GCV), cytosine deaminase (CD) of *E. coli* with 5-fluorocytosine (5-FC), cytochrome P450 with cyclophosphamide/ifosfamide (CPA/IFA), and nitroreductase with CB1954 Gene silencing: siRNA	*Lactococcus, Streptococcus, Bifidobacterium, Escherichia, Salmonella, Clostridia*
Bacterial oncolytic therapy	Bacterial spores	*Clostridium, Escherichia*
Bacteria as immunotherapeutic agents	Expressing antigen DNA vaccines	*Salmonella, Bifidobacterium, Escherichia,*
Bacterial toxins	Protein toxins inhibiting cellular processes	*Campylobacter, Helicobacter, Pseudomonas, Stapylococcus, Bordetella*

drug. Other mechanisms involving the transfer of the eukaryotic expression vectors into cancerous cells, expression of the gene-silencing siRNAs, cytokines, tumor antigen that can inflict the trigger of the immune system have also been investigated. The new strategies for the expression of various anti-tumor agents are increasing due to the development in the system biology and recent advances in metagenomics.

3.1 Recombinant Bacteria

The genetic engineering techniques have exhibited the insertion of the plasmid vectors that can be encoded as proteins in the form of antigens, anti-bodies, cytokines, and enzymes. The expression can be changed by introducing the promoters into live bacteria. Those nonpathogenic bacteria are termed as GRAS ('generally regarded as safe') bacteria. *Lactococcus lactis* has been engineered widely for protein production. In phase I clinical trial, *L. lactis* has been used for the delivery of the anti-inflammatory cytokine interleukin-10 (IL-10) to intestinal mucosa as a treatment module in the patients suffering from inflammatory bowel disease (Yoo et al. 2011). The commensals, for example, *Streptococcus gordonii*, have a capability to colonize mucosal surfaces in the oral, nasal, and vaginal cavity. It has been engineered to act as a vehicle for the production and delivery of biologically active proteins.

Bacteria have likewise been effectively utilized as the vehicle carrying the vectors that can express the RNA interference (RNAi) for the disease treatment. *Salmonella* strains have been engineered to deliver plasmid siRNA to tumors and smother in vivo tumor growth. The recombinant strains have siRNAs for silencing the multidrug-resistant genes and act as signal transducers. Few strains have activator of transcription-specific siRNAs to inhibit the growth of the tumor. Another bacterium, *Escherichia coli,* has been engineered to carry vector with siRNAs and has been the successful model (in vitro and in vivo) of gene silencing in human colon cancer. It has been reported that expression of transkingdom RNAi plasmid encodes proteins such as invasion for cellular internalization, listeriolysin O for endosomal escape, and short hairpin RNA against the cancer gene, catenin β1.

In the preclinical models, *Salmonella typhimurium* has been engineered to express interleukin-2 (IL-2) for the treatment of liver tumors. Cytokine IL-2 has the prestige of extensively studied bacterially delivered cytokine. The study has shown that oral administration of *Salmonella* expressing IL-2 can function prophylactically and prevents tumor formation. However, there is a limited success with these microbes due to the systemic toxicities.

VNP20009 has been engineered to express therapeutic proteins, such as TNF-α and platelet factor 4 fragment. *S. typhimurium*, (SL3261) an auxotroph, has been engineered to the introduction of cytomegalovirus (CMV) promoter controlling the expression of the cloned genes ofhIL-12, hGM-CSF, mIL-12, and mGM-CSF. In the mice models bearing Lewis lung carcinomas, oral administration of *Salmonella* expressing mGM-CSF or mGM-CSF plus mIL-12 has shown significant tumor regression. *Clostridium acetobutylicum* has been engineered to express functional TNF-α and has been reported to kill cancerous cells through apoptosis in adenocarcinomas.

3.2 Bacterial Directed Enzyme Prodrug Therapy

This technique beats the inadmissible adverse effects of bacterial treatment and utilizes anaerobic bacteria transformed with an enzyme capable of converting a non-poisonous prodrug into a toxic medication for tumors. In the enzyme prodrug system, bacteria can multiply in the necrotic and hypoxic parts of the tumor, thereby exclusively expressing drug-activating enzyme in the tumor. A nontoxic prodrug is administered systemically which can act as a substrate of the exogenous enzyme and is metabolized to the lethal medication for a tumor. A few enzyme/prodrug systems are accessible. The most extensively studied pairs are herpes simplex virus thymidine kinase (HSV-TK) with ganciclovir (GCV), cytosine deaminase (CD) of *E. coli* with 5-fluorocytosine (5-FC), cytochrome P450 with cyclophosphamide/ifosfamide (CPA/IFA), and nitroreductase with CB1954 (Lehouritis et al. 2013).

CD-5FC system is the well-studied enzyme of gene directed enzyme prodrug therapy. It catalyzes the deamination of cytosine into uracil and has been studied as a member of the pyrimidine nucleotide salvage pathway. It has the focus on only one prodrug, 5-FC. The wide use of the 5-FU in the chemotherapy has shown various adverse events because of the high dosage. The CD converts the 5-FC into 5-FU and toxicity is directed only to the tumor cells. The resulted 5-FU can be further converted by cellular enzymes into potent pyrimidine antimetabolites that can trigger the death of the cancerous cells. CD/5-FC therapy has been studied in a wide variety of in vitro and in vivo animal models of cancers. It has been shown that MDA-MB-231 breast carcinoma cells transfected with *E. coli* CD were 1000-fold more sensitive to 5-FC in comparison with the control. CD can be effectively cloned and expressed in the *Clostridium*, and expression was improved altogether by the vascular focusing on operators (combretastatin A-4 phosphate). This improvement might be because of the extension of the expression in the necrotic range inside the tumors.

Various clinical trials using CD/5-FC system have reported limited success. A phase I clinical trial conducted for patients with breast cancer has shown safety with significant levels of erB-2 suicide gene expression by the use of the tumor-specific erbB-2 promoter. As of now, there are three clinical trials in progress. One is for treatment of recurrent high-grade glioma (NCT01172964), whereas two others are for solid tumors (NCT01562626) and for malignant brain tumor (NCT01470794) (Zhang et al. 2015).

Nitroreductases (NR) metabolize aromatic nitrogroups to hydroxylamines by generating massive electronic change that causes cytotoxicity. It is oxygen-insensitive flavin-mononucleotide nitroreductase found in *E. coli*. The most successful prodrug used for therapy in conjunction with nitroreductase is 5-aziridinyl-2,4-dinitrobenzamide (CB 1954, or Prolarix), which is the prototype of the dinitrobenzamide family of prodrugs. The metabolites of CB1954 are potent alkylating agents, which kill both dividing and non-diving tumor cells. The metabolites are highly cell-permeable which showed a strong bystander effect for killing the adjacent tumor cells. The efficacy of this NR-CB1954 system has been demonstrated in a few clinical trials for treatment of liver and prostate cancers.

There have been clinical trials with the use of the *Salmonella* vector having expression of NR and CD in the diseased patients. *S. typhimurium* having VNP20009 vector has been engineered to *E. coli* CD for TAPET (Tumor Amplified Protein Expression Therapy). Although there is clinical safety of *S. typhimurium* as shown in the phase I trial, there is little effect on the recurrence of the cancer in the human trials. Nonetheless, there is still cause for optimism with further improvements in genetic technologies for the species (Liu et al. 2014).

4 Bacterial Oncolytic Therapy

The oncolytic approach for the cancer treatment utilizes the competent bacteria with replicative behavior in the tumor tissues the bacteria can replicate and kill the tumor. Therapeutic trials involving *Clostridium* spores rely on the oncolytic activity of the bacteria. Administration of the clostridia spores through intravenous pathway produces oncolytic effects in the preclinical and the clinical studies. Marked lysis was observed with the *C. histolyticum* spores and with the spores of *Clostridium sporogenes*.

The use of the spores of the anaerobic bacteria has greater advantage in the bacterial therapy in cancer, as these spores can survive the hypoxia and the necrosis conditions of the tumor. The spores become viable in the tumor microenvironment and hence can proliferate in the tumor. After the lysis of the tumor, these bacteria cannot survive the oxygen-rich environment; therefore, these are the best surgical scissors for the tumor treatment with less toxicity and complete destruction of the tumor cells.

There is requirement of the genetic engineering of the *clostridium* species with repetitive screens to enhance the colonization of the tumor. Various recombinant strains such as *Clostridium oncolyticum*, *Clostridium beijerinckii* (*acetobutylicum*), *Clostridium tetani*, *C. oncolyticum* (*sporogenes*), and *C. novyi–NT* have been utilized for the tumor treatment.

Bacterial spores have additionally been exploited as delivery agents for cytotoxic peptides, anticancer agents, therapeutic proteins as well as vectors for gene therapy. It has also been shown that *S. typhimurium* A1 strain can grow easily in prostate cancer cells and kill the cancer cells by nuclear destruction and cell death. Hence, this property of replication and finally colonization produces minimum toxicity.

5 Bacterial Toxins

Toxins have been used for the cancer treatment since time immemorial. Bacterial toxins inhibit the protein synthesis by ADP ribosylation of elongation factor 2. The bacterial toxins have greater impact on the cellular processes controlling growth, proliferation, apoptosis, and differentiation. Bacterial toxins are capable of binding with the cell surface antigen, thereby generating the immune response (Rosadi et al. 2016). Diphtheria toxin (DT) binds to the surface of cells expressing the heparin-binding epidermal growth factors such as growth factor (HB-EGF) precursor forming DT-HB-EGF. Endocytosis of this DT-HB-EGF through clathrin-vesicles prompts several posttranslational modifications resulting in a catalytically active toxin, called DT fragment A. DT fragment A can ribosylate EF-2 leading to halting of protein synthesis with subsequent cell lysis and/or induction of apoptosis (Frankel et al. 2001). Similarly, *Pseudomonas* exotoxin (PE) A is also known to catalytically ribosylate EF-2 and hence inhibits protein synthesis. It has been shown in the mice that i.v. injection of 0.3 μg of this toxin has lethal cytotoxicity, thereby making it a potential contender for the targeted cancer therapy.

Clostridium perfringens enterotoxin (CPE) produced by *C. perfringens* type A strain causes gastroenteritis. The C terminal domain of endotoxin has high affinity binding to the CPE receptor (CPE-R) and the N-terminal domain causes cytotoxicity. It has been demonstrated that purified endotoxin can kill colon, breast, gastric, and pancreatic tumor cells. Cholera toxins have also been shown to be cytotoxic. Some bacterial toxins (alfa-toxins from *Stapylococcus aureus*, AC-toxin from *Bordetella pertussis,* and shiga like toxins) are being investigated in the cancer cell lines. These toxins have shown an increased cytotoxicity and triggering apoptosis. It has been reported that *Botulinum* neurotoxin (BoNT) has the capability of opening tumor vessels. It can be used for enhancing the effects of the radiotherapy and chemotherapy on the cancer cells. BoNT effect on the tumor microenvironment shows the indirect action for the cytotoxic effect.

Bacterial toxins may be ideal for the fusing with the ligands because these are expressed in the bacteria as single chains with binding domains that can be exchanged for a ligand in the tumor. This strategy can be completed by deliberately eliminating the binding to the toxin receptors by conjugation with cell-binding proteins (monoclonal antibodies or growth factors) that can selectively kill cancer cells. A wide variety of ligands such as IL-3, IL-4, G-CSF, transferrin, EGF, and vascular endothelial growth factor (VEGF) have been conjugated to DT to study the effect on the tumors. There have been clinical trials involving transferrin-DT conjugate (Tf-CRM) and DT-EGF inpatients of brain tumor and metastatic carcinomas, respectively. Similarly, various antibodies and ligands have been conjugated to PE. Conjugation of IL-4, IL-13, monoclonal antibody-recognizing a carbohydrate antigen Lewis Y, (Mab B3), and transforming growth factor (TGF-α) to PE has been studied in the clinical trials.

6 Bacteria as Immunotherapeutic Agents

Immune system is the defense of life. Immune therapy is an effective and emerging strategy for cancer treatment. Immunology concentrates on the killing of tumor cells through direct or indirect attack of the effector immune cells; B cells with antibody production, T cells, Natural Killer cells, dendritic cells. Malignant tissues have the system to evade the immune system. An insight into the regulation of processes leads to immune-based therapies for cancer. To evade the immune system, tumor cells can secrete various cytokines that evade the immune system. Bacteria can be utilized for the production of immune-upregulating cytokines that can attract the lymphocytes (Nelson et al. 2015). It has been demonstrated that attenuated *S. typhimurium* can infect the cancerous cells in several murine trials triggering immune response. There was significant tumor reduction due to local bacterial expression or expression of immune-stimulating molecules IL-18, Fas ligand. It has also been reported that IL-2-encoding *Salmonella* organisms have shown better suppression of the tumors than the wild types. Preclinical studies with *Bifidobacteria* expressing granulocyte colony-stimulating factor (GCSF) resulted in superior anti-tumor effects. The immune response resulted in the killings of the tumor cells.

Another strategy is the use of DNA vaccines that helps to sensitize the immune system for the specific antigen expressed by tumor cells. DNA vaccines have shown significant efficacy in preclinical and clinical trials. The tumor antigenic DNA is introduced into the bacteria such as *Salmonella* and *Listeria* that is specifically expressed and triggered the immune cells, thereby showing immunity in the animal models. Vaccination strategies stimulate the required response by generating enhanced immune reaction for the tumor. Bacteria that can raise the immune response by them have been the ideal candidate for the delivery of DNA vaccines.

Attenuated *S. typhimurium* introduced with human tumor endothelial marker 8 (TEM8) DNA gene has been reported to generate CD8 cytotoxic T-cell response in the animal models. *Salmonella* is taken up by the monocytes in the intestine for lysis and for the relaese of the vector thereby triggering the immune reaction. A recombinant strain of attenuated *S. typhimurium* expressing a gene encoding LIGHT has been reported to inhibit the growth of primary tumors in mouse models with lesser toxicity (Ruan et al. 2009).

Systemic administration of *C. novyi-NT* spores has elicited the inflammation and the leukocytosis by expressing various cytokines such as IL-6, IL-2, and GS-CSF. These cytokines can further attract the neutrophils. Inflammation leads to the production of the reactive oxygen species, thereby producing the oxidative stress and killing of tumors.

Attenuated and live strains of *Listeria* have been used for expressing a broad range of tumor antigens. The expressions of the oncogenes such as Her-2/neu, Melanoma Associated Antigen, and PSA, have helped in the enhanced immune response. A vaccine strain of *Listeria monocytogenes* (Lm-NP) with the nucleoprotein (NP) from influenza strain A/PR8/34 has shown the regression of tumors. Patients suffering from metastatic cervical cancer have been intravenously administrated with attenuated *L. monocytogenes* expressing HPV16 E7 in phase I clinical trial. There was 30 % tumor reduction in the overall survival with some flu-like symptoms and fever-related hypertension in some patients. This successful trial has shown the safety and efficacy of Listeria vectors in cancer patients (Wood et al. 2008). Another successful story is related to the bovis Bacillus Calmette-Guérin (BCG-CWS). The cell wall skeleton of the Mycobacterium has been used for enhancing the immune system in the cancer patients. BCG/CWS has also been known for the radio sensitizing effect on colon cancer cells through the induction of autophagic cell death. The results were promising for in vitro and in vivo studies. Hence, (BCG-CWS) can be therapeutic strategy for enhancing immune response with the promising lesser toxicity with non-virulent bacteria. BCG the most successful bacterial agent so far is used specifically for the treatment of superficial bladder cancer. It has been reported that tumor cells can be killed by preventing the new blood vessel formation of the cutting of the nutrient supply. The transfer of the anti-angiogenic genes endostatin and thrombospondin can thereby easily kill tumors. Transfer of endostatin from *Salmonella* has shown the reduced microvessel density, diminished vascular endothelial growth factor (VEGF) expression, and slowed tumor growth in mice. However, there was minimal effect on direct administration of endostatin to patients. Similar strategies have been used for the reduction of tumor growth using genes encoding for TRAIL, SMAC, and FASL.

7 Bacteria in Combination Therapy

The use of the bacteria or the specifically engineered bacteria along with the conventional therapies is termed as combination bacteriolytic therapy (COBALT). Conventional chemotherapeutic agents such as docetaxel, mitomycin C, vinorelbine, and dolastatin-10 have been supplemented with *C. novyi-NT* spores. It has shown significant anti-tumor properties with serious adverse reactions. *C. novyi* has also been investigated into combination with other conventional modalities such as radiotherapy and radioimmunotherapy in the experimental tumor models with the progressive results. It has the potential of combined multi-modality approaches to future cancer therapies. Due to the membrane-disrupting property of the *C. novyi-NT*, it has been exploited to enhance the release of liposome-encapsulated drugs within tumors. This strain has also been used in combination with anti-microtubule agents, thereby decreasing the vascularized regions and enhancing the effects of the drugs.

8 Conclusions and Future Perspective

Bacterial therapy has shown a greater promise in the intense and the diverse field of cancer treatment due to its potential to regress the tumor completely and its ability to deliver the therapeutic products. Bacteria have been investigated by various means for the cancer treatment modalities. Live or attenuated bacteria with different vectors have emerged as potential strategies for the cancer management. The genetically engineered microbes have shown the lesser toxicity for the normal cells and better efficacy for the treatment. Bacteria have been engineered to carry the plasmids having the gene of interest that can be directed to the tumors. These alterations produce the mutant strain that has the capacity to express the anticancer agents. Attenuated *Salmonella* with VNP20009 and TAPET-CD have been investigated successfully in phase I clinical trials in cancer patients. Facultative anaerobes have shown to be colonizing the tumors by complex mechanisms but showing greater efficacy. Bacterial therapy in combination with the conventional modalities has shown the better efficacy of the treatment as well as better quality of life for the patients suffering from spectrum of cancer. Bioengineering of bacteria can be helpful in creating a new modality for the cancer therapy. There is a need for the new investigations to study the better use of the bacteria in the cancer treatment.

References

Forbes NS (2010) Engineering the perfect (bacterial) cancer therapy. Nat Rev Cancer 10:785–794

Frahm M, Felgner S, Kocijancic D et al (2015) Efficiency of conditionally attenuated *Salmonella enterica* serovar Typhimurium in bacterium-mediated tumor therapy. mBio 6(2): e00254-15

Frankel AE, Rossi P, Kuzel TM et al (2001) Diphtheria fusion protein therapy of chemoresistant malignancies. Curr Cancer Drug Targets 2:19–36

Hanahan D, Weinberg RA (2011) Hallmarks of cancer: the next generation. Cell 144:646–674

Lehouritis P, Springer C, Tangney M (2013) Bacterial-directed enzyme prodrug therapy. J Control Release 170:120–131

Liu S, Xu X, Zeng X et al (2014) Tumor-targeting bacterial therapy: a potential treatment for oral cancer. Oncol Lett 8:2359–2366

Nelson MH, Diven MA, Huff LW et al (2015) Harnessing the microbiome to enhance cancer immunotherapy. J Immunol Res. doi:10.1155/2015/368736

Patyar S, Joshi R, Byrav DS et al (2010) Bacteria in cancer therapy: a novel experimental strategy. J Biomed Sci 17:21–29

Roberts NJ, Zhang L, Janku F et al (2014) Intratumoral injection of *Clostridium novyi*-NT spores induces antitumor responses. SciTransl Med. doi:10.1126/scitranslmed.3008982

Rosadi F, Fiorentini C, Fabbri A (2016) Bacterial protein toxins in human cancers. Pathog Dis. doi:10.1093/femspd/ftv105

Ruan Z, Yang Z, Wang Y (2009) DNA vaccine against tumor endothelial marker 8 inhibits tumor angiogenesis and growth. J Immunother 32:486–491

Wood LM, Guirnalda PD, Seavey MM et al (2008) Cancer immunotherapy using *Listeria monocytogenes* and listerial virulence factors. Immunol Res 42:233–245

Yoo JW, Irvine DJ, Discher DE et al (2011) Bio-inspired, bioengineered and biomimetic drug delivery carriers. Nat Rev Drug Discov 10:521–535

Zhang J, Kale V, Chen M (2015) Gene-directed enzyme prodrug therapy. AAPS J 17:102–110

FSC
www.fsc.org
MIX
Papier | Fördert gute Waldnutzung
FSC® C083411

Kolibri 360 GmbH
Ferdinand-Jühlke-Straße 7
99095 Erfurt, Deutschland
produktsicherheit@kolibri360.de